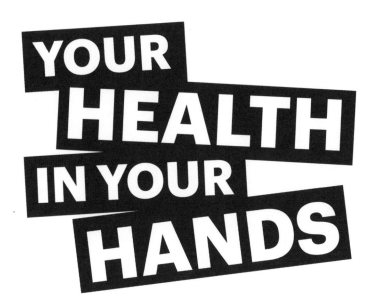

YOUR HEALTH IN YOUR HANDS

AN ESSENTIAL HANDBOOK TO FUTUREPROOF YOUR HEALTH

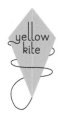

yellow
kite

Photography by Nassima Rothacker

Doctor Emeka

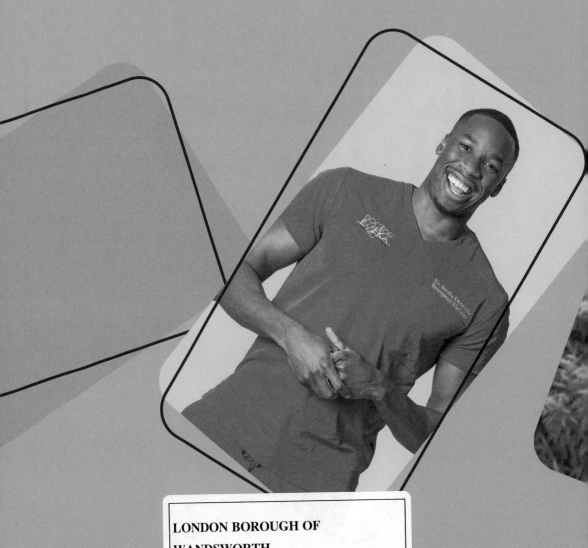

YOUR HEALTH IN YOUR HANDS

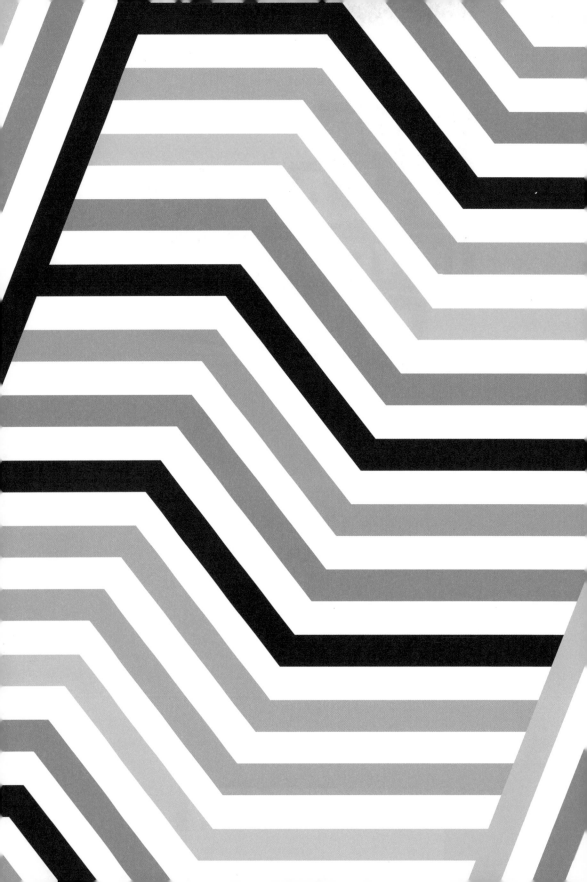

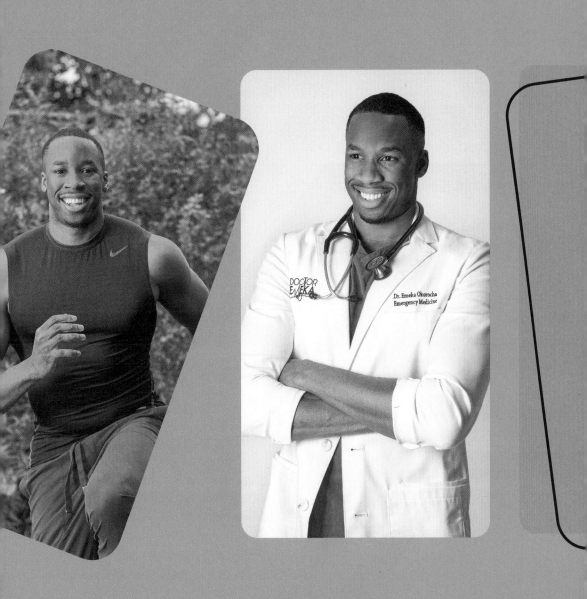

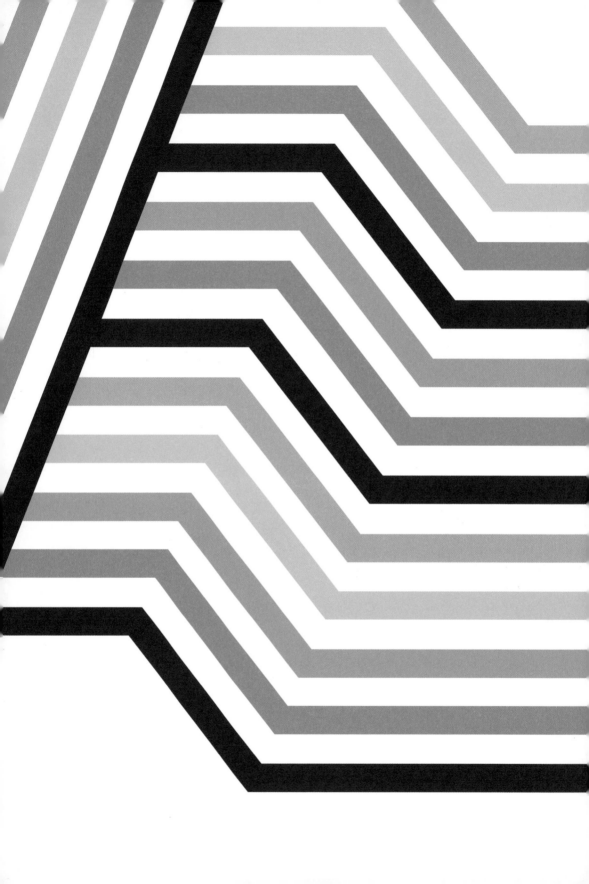

MY NAME IS DR. EMEKA OKOROCHA, AND I WANT TO DO MY BEST FOR YOUR HEALTH.

I want to know what your problem is.
I want to know where it hurts.
I want to know how long it's been going on.
I want to know what makes it better.
I want to know if it's happened before.
I want to know if anything has changed.
My name is Dr. Emeka Okorocha,
and I want to do my best for your health.

DR.

EMEKA

I was born in Nigeria 28 years ago and my family emigrated to the UK in search of a better education and quality of life for myself and my older sister when we were just toddlers. My grandfather was king of a province, leaving my dad (his first son) and myself (also the first son) as princes. In our family, as first sons, we have the same initials and it always makes me feel so very proud to share this legacy and heritage from the country of my birth with my dad and grandfather. Though I've spent most of my life here in the UK, I want to one day go back to Nigeria and take all the lessons I've learnt to help better the health and emergency care system over there, in my much-loved homeland.

WHERE IT ALL BEGAN

Being fit and active have always come very naturally to me. As a young boy, I had lots of energy and just wanted to run everywhere as fast as possible and play with my friends. I loved the idea of competition, and playing sports was my passion.

Whenever my parents asked me what I wanted to be when I grew up, my reply would usually be: 'I'm not sure yet, but I want to do all the good I can. I want to make a change and I want to be known.' I always assumed this would be from my sporting accolades, but as I got older it was evident that my passion for medicine and the human body was growing alongside my zest for sports and activity.

Medicine is in my blood. My father is a doctor and so was my grandfather. Being born into a family of medics is great on the one hand because it means you have access to a lot of information about your future career. However, it also means there is a lot of pressure on your back. But it has been such an inspiration to see what my father has achieved and, from my father and grandfather, I heard about the life-saving changes doctors and surgeons made in people's lives and it both fascinated

and inspired me. I thought that I could make some of those changes and differences to people's lives too, and so I pursued a career in medicine. Medicine is such a broad, complex career that there is bound to be a domain to suit your lifestyle and personality if it's something that appeals to you.

During my first year of medical school, we learnt about social medicine and the combination of general health and the human body, which only cemented my mission to help others improve their health through lifestyle changes.

I have worked in a number of different specialties over the years, but I am someone who likes a fast-paced challenge and so I knew that emergency medicine, where I work now, was the way forward for me as I felt it was where I could make the most impact. Working in emergency departments has given me the opportunity and time to expand my medical knowledge and use the skills I've gained to educate others – being a doctor is the best thing ever and I can't think of a more fulfilling job.

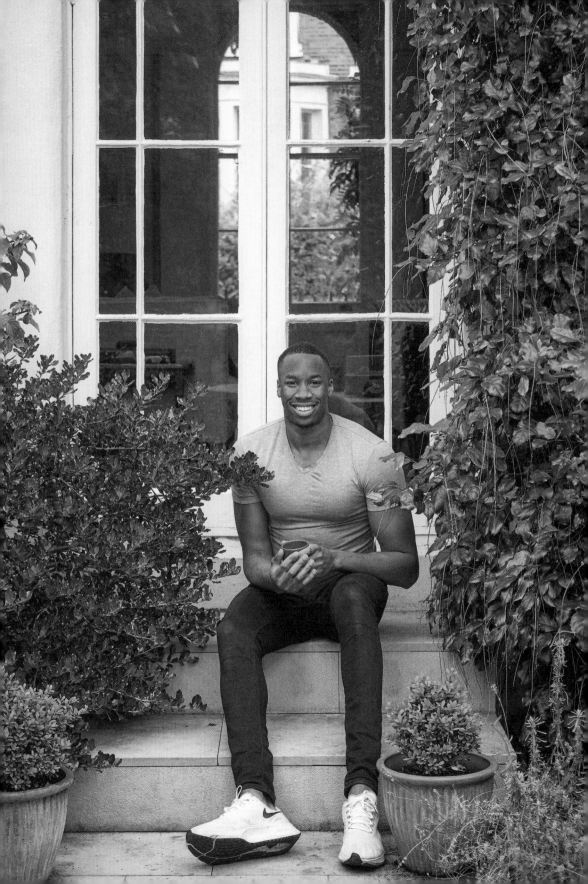

MY
MISS
ION

LEARN
EDUCATE
EMPOWER
INSPIRE
CREATE
CHANGE

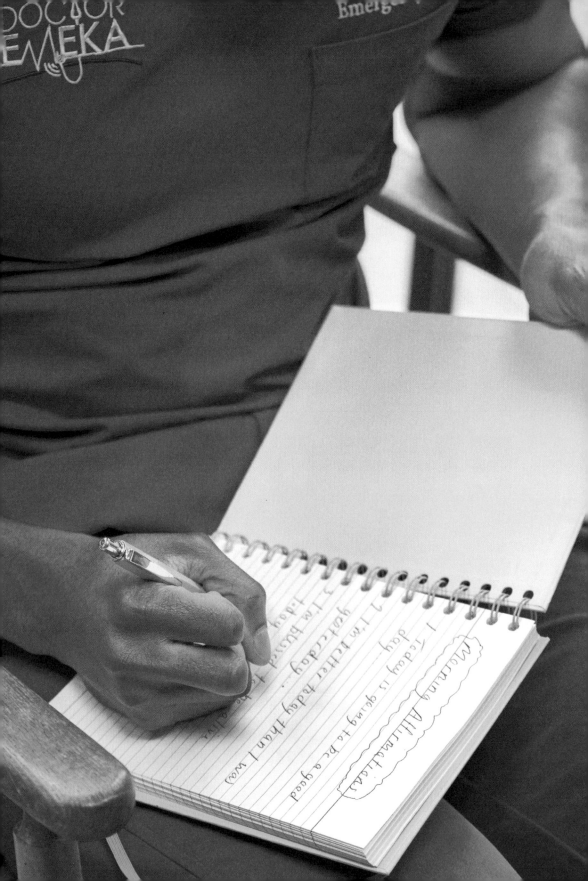

Why this book?

One of the reasons I've written this book is due to what I've witnessed as a doctor. When you see people coming into A&E, it opens your eyes to what can manifest if you don't take care of your health. I try to take a learning point from each case and, alongside helping the patient, I look at how I can better myself and my own health so I can educate patients to better theirs.

Working in A&E I am obviously involved in dealing with life and death emergencies on a daily basis – and being able to spring into action to help save people's lives in a heartbeat is an amazing privilege and a wonderful feeling. One other thing I absolutely love about being at the front face of patient care is the opportunity to give the patients I see simple health advice on a range of different topics to help them live longer – including how they can improve their mental health, sleep better, eat better... the list goes on – which will help aid their recovery and hopefully keep them out of hospital in the future. I'm a firm believer that small changes can make a big difference over time. So in this book I'm going to be dropping lots of those health hacks I share with my patients, showing you how you can improve your overall health with a bunch of simple methods and start kicking them into action like second nature.

It's a shame that a lot of the patients I see in A&E haven't taken their health seriously for a number of years and have developed preventable chronic diseases as a result. For many of them, this leads to an untimely downfall. We know that people are at high risk of developing serious illnesses if they have medical problems like cardiovascular disease, diabetes, chronic respiratory disease, cancer and other comorbidities. The silver lining is that we can prevent many of these, and I'll discuss how in this book.

Young people in particular tend to be under the impression that they are invincible and that their health isn't a major priority. However, the small habits we have when we are young make a drastic difference to our health as we age; these tiny incremental lifestyle factors build up to the bigger picture as time rolls on. It can be really hard to see the benefits, or conversely the damaging impacts, in the moment or 'in the now' – so I want this book to encourage young readers to start taking care of their health as early as possible. Many of my older patients suffering from various chronic diseases always say that they wish they'd known how important their habits were when they were younger. Once you are more aware of the risk factors that can cause certain diseases you can tackle them appropriately and ensure you take measures to better your own health – such as getting active, losing weight, improving your diet and adopting a healthier lifestyle.

MY TIKTOK JOURNEY

During the coronavirus lockdown in 2020 I started a TikTok platform making fun, informative videos about healthcare and how people could keep safe from Covid-19. Living alone in London during the pandemic, TikTok was initially a great outlet to provide me with some stress relief from the emotional strain of everything I was seeing and dealing with on a daily basis in the hospital Covid wards. But I soon began to see how fun and creative social media could be and I realised I could actually use this app to inform people, not only about the pandemic but about health and medicine generally, as well as social issues, myth-busting common misconceptions and countering misinformation, while shaking a leg and busting some of my funniest, trendiest dance moves! TikTok became my world stage to share healthcare messages and empowering knowledge far and wide. This book is an extension of that content, and is packed with tips to help everyone identify and modify the behaviours that may be harming their health. Alongside this, I also want to continue my myth-busting mission. We live in a social media world full of information about how to live well, and there is so much confusing and conflicting advice out there. I'm therefore going to lay bare some of the medical myths that I've come across in practice and on the internet, debunking those that are solely myths and unravelling those that actually have some truth to them.

GOING VIRAL

Sometimes I use social media to highlight other stuff I feel strongly about. For example, during 2020, as well as the coronavirus pandemic, we were faced with a lot of global social issues. With the well-known death of George Floyd (rest in peace) we were all exposed to just how much police brutality and racism is present in America and around the world. Unfortunately, as a Black man in the UK, I've also been subjected to racism and prejudice in a number of different forms.

Individuals in Black, Asian and minority ethnic communities around the UK and the world have been facing racism and discrimination for years, and I wanted to highlight just how important it was that people knew about this, so that we can make an adequate change and strive to be anti-racist as a society. So I made a video of myself in my hoodie and also in my scrubs and contrasted how people see me in both. 'If you celebrate me in my scrubs, don't hate me in my hoodie' was the message I wanted to send. I don't want to be clapped for and celebrated when I am wearing my scrubs and PPE, only to be racially profiled for wearing a simple hoodie. I am the same man in both the scrubs and the hoodie and shouldn't be discriminated against just because of how I dress. However, that's a reality for many people of colour. Hopefully that video, and others I made, can highlight these issues so we can solve them and eradicate them for future generations. Don't love us just when it's trendy or convenient. Love us when it's hard; when you may be criticised; when you may be scared or embarrassed. That's when we really will feel you stand with us.

Health and well-being is not all about your physical health. As a doctor in A&E, I saw the effects of Covid-19 – not just physically but mentally too – as lockdown caused untold damage to people's mental health and outlook. If the pandemic has taught us anything it is how key it is to take our mental health seriously, and do everything we can to reduce stress and boost a positive mindset and mood. I know it's so hard to find motivation to do the things that you know will ease your mind when you're in a low place, and you can't see the benefits instantly, but it makes a whole lot of difference if you can start building healthy daily routines or find tools that you know work for you which you can fall back on in tough times. We should be trying to open up to people and form strong relationships with friends and loved ones. We should also be trying to take regular breaks from work or routines that cause us stress so that we can help reduce any overwhelming feelings or anxiety. And so this book will also show you ways to maintain your mental health, keeping your mood and mind at the most optimal level possible.

I'M NOT TRYING TO SCARE YOU, BUT...

Now I'm normally one for complete positivity. And generally everything I say, and my mindset, tends to be very optimistic. However, sometimes we have to be realistic to understand just how important our health is. And part of this is knowing where things can go wrong if we don't take it seriously.

I have seen things as a doctor which have really shaken me up and it's made me realise how fragile our bodies and minds are – it's made me even more passionate about getting important, responsible healthcare information out there for people to consume. So there are going to be a number of negative statistics in this book; this isn't to scare you, but to make you more mindful of the realities of staying healthy. Sometimes to change our lives we need stressors – push and pull factors – to really make a difference. Pull factors could be looking and feeling better and having a better quality of life. And then push factors could be circumstances you want to escape from and situations you want to avoid.

As medical professionals, we have to make life-changing decisions on a daily basis. What we do every day can make a real difference to people's lives, but we also understand the impact that potential mistakes can have on people's futures. We have to work fast, but we also have to work smart and as part of a team. Across the brilliant NHS in general we all try to work with the same objective and the same goal: to get the patient better and provide the best care we can. You'll see throughout the book that I discuss some of the cases I've seen in A&E. I feel this is my way of giving back to the community to show just how your health and lifestyle can impact your life. All the cases I describe are real, but have been anonymised for patient confidentiality. However intense they may seem, this is stuff I've seen and these are real stories about patients I've treated.

YOUR
HEALTH
IN YOUR
HANDS

None of us know what's going to happen with the passing of time, but managing your health now in the present will give you more control and a better chance of staying fitter and healthier for longer in the future. This book will help you to 'futureproof' your health with tools you can utilise to change your life in the long term, giving you the best chance of fighting off chronic diseases and acute illnesses such as infections, and essentially help you live a longer, healthier, more fulfilling life.

I want to equip you with preventative healthcare advice that you can easily understand and digest to enable you to make short-term decisions that could have an amazing, positive impact on your long-term health.

We all have a responsibility, especially now in these unprecedented times, to look after ourselves and encourage our loved ones to do the same. This book – like your health – is now in your hands. I hope it empowers you with accessible and actionable advice for better health and self-care to help you have a brighter future.

'I want to equip you with preventative healthcare advice that you can easily understand and digest.'

DR. EMEKA'S MINUTES THAT MATTER:
The morning routine

Sometimes I feel people don't understand just how important mornings are; a morning routine creates the fundamental template – the building blocks – for a better, brighter day. That's why, even when it feels like time is short, I make sure mine gets me buzzed and motivated to achieve everything I need to do... those morning minutes really do matter.

GIVE THANKS

One of the first things I do when I wake up is take a minute to give thanks to God for a new day. In my profession, it's difficult to take life for granted because you see so many people who don't have the opportunity to get up every day or who get up but are in pain or in circumstances that many wouldn't even be able to fathom. I'm religious by background, though I appreciate that many people are not. If you don't follow a particular faith, it may still be useful to shout out or speak out about all of the things that you're thankful for in life, such as your family, your friends and your health. This puts you in a positive mindset, and studies have shown that when we express gratitude, or even receive it, our brains release dopamine and serotonin which are our natural antidepressants – basically the chemicals in our brain which enhance our mood and immediately make us feel fuzzy inside.

Gratitude is a powerful human emotion which is known to provide optimism, reduce stress and anxiety, and help us feel better. Taking just a few minutes each morning to feel thankful and grateful will help you to stay optimistic and appreciate everything you go through during the day.

USE AFFIRMATIONS

After giving thanks, I love to go through affirmations – usually phrases I have written down in a notebook that I read from every morning. I say really positive things about what's going well for me in life and what's going well with my family. This puts me in the right frame of mind to start my day and significantly boosts my mood. I will often say out loud things like, 'I'm really successful and good fortune follows me. I have an amazing support network. I live such a happy life. My health is as good as it's ever been.'

I feel that affirmations give you and your subconscious mind a vision of yourself, and their power brings good fortune towards you.

- **'I'm thankful to be alive.'**
- **'Yesterday's lessons become today's practice.'**
- **'Today is going to be a good day.'**
- **'I want to impact someone's life today.'**
- **'Today is going to be a productive day.'**
- **'I'm going to have fun today.'**
- **'Today the world needs me at my best.'**
- **'Today is another opportunity to make myself great.'**
- **'Today's tasks will bring me closer to my goals.'**
- **'Today I'm going to learn something new.'**

MEDITATE

Another good morning hack is to meditate and clear your mind for just one minute. Spend a minute not trying to think about too much. Try not to distract yourself with anything – just concentrate on your breathing and your heart rate and simply relax. This works very well for people who get morning anxiety or who have too many tasks for the day and don't know how they will complete them. A massive amount of illness is actually stress-related, so by doing this every day you're likely to keep yourself healthier and happier.

GET OUTSIDE

Sometimes when my alarm goes off, I feel very lethargic or demotivated and want to go back to sleep. When this happens, I like to act fast before I can allow myself to hit the 'snooze' button. So I leave my house and go for a 10-minute walk to get refreshed. Often just getting out of bed, breathing some fresh air into my lungs and allowing the light to hit my eyes lets my body know that it's time to get up and get going.

MAKE A PLAN

Another great morning ritual is to plan and strategise how you are going to attack the day, possibly with an organiser, calendar or to-do list so you can prioritise tasks.

I usually do this after I've asked myself the questions below. This makes the day more manageable and less stressful and helps you organise your life much better. If I'm on the go, I even use the 'notes' app on my phone and add to it throughout the day. Ticking off or working through wins cuts through the noise, makes you feel less overwhelmed and helps get things straight.

QUESTION YOURSELF

Another very important thing I do every morning is take a minute to ask myself an important question. I make the questions profound enough to make me think and be impactful, which helps me determine what I'm actually going to do for the day and how it's going to help me get to where I need to be.

1. **What do you plan to achieve today?**
2. **How are you going to impact someone's life today?**
3. **How are the tasks you're doing going to get you to your goals?**
4. **How will you make yourself great today?**
5. **If today was your last day, would you be doing this?**
6. **What are you planning on learning today?**
7. **How can you be better than yesterday?**
8. **How will you make today productive?**
9. **Who's likely to help you to achieve your goals today?**
10. **How is your today going to impact your tomorrow?**

STRETCH

Getting yourself ready for the day physically is just as important as preparing yourself mentally. Before breakfast, I like to to do a full body stretch from top to toe to make sure I loosen all my joints. This gets you ready for any exercise during the day, can help to safeguard against injuries and even prevent long-lasting chronic joint and muscle pain.

MORNING STRETCH

1. **Squat down with your feet shoulder-width apart. Put your elbows on your knees with your back straight and hold for five deep breaths.**
2. **Walk your hands forward into 'downward dog', hold for five breaths.**
3. **Move your right leg forward into a lunge, move your right hand inside your foot and rotate to point your left hand towards the sky. Repeat on the other side.**
4. **Stand up straight and take three deep breaths, bringing both arms up to the sky with each breath.**

HYDRATE

An important habit that you can implement into your morning routine is to make sure you get a good amount of water. Often when we sleep we can lose a lot of fluid from sweat and become dehydrated from just breathing, especially if we sleep with our mouths open. Dehydration and lack of fluid can lead to us feeling lethargic, having headaches and even feeling a bit confused in the morning, and it has a profound effect on our mental performance throughout the day. So it's imperative that when we wake up we make sure that we drink a good glass of fresh water.

LOOK TO THE FUTURE

Taking a minute to cross off your achievements or reflect is a very powerful technique to have you looking forward to the future. Whether yesterday has gone really well for you or very badly, it's important to focus on the present. Take away any positives or lessons from the previous day, then acknowledge that it has now gone and is something of the past. This type of thinking keeps your goals in the forefront of your mind.

One-minute health hack

SELF-REFLECTION

For one minute sit and ask yourself these five questions. Try to answer each one honestly and openly.

1. **Am I truly happy?**
2. **If yes, why? If no, why not?**
3. **How could I make myself feel better?**
4. **Is there anything bothering me right now?**
5. **What steps could I take to do something about it?**

Answering these questions every morning will help you reflect, and slowly and regularly identify life factors which may be bothering you or affecting your mood on a day-to-day basis, thus hopefully preventing things from building up and causing long-term mental health issues.

And there you have it! You're ready to start the day!

HEALTHY VIII

HOW TO LIVE LONGER:
The basics revisited

MOTIVATION

Rather than a mandatory drag after the weekend, treat Mondays as an opportunity to start a new day in a new week and be better at your craft than you were last week. Start your week with this mindset and you're bound to be maximising your potential in no time!

Life will eventually come to an end for all of us. But who doesn't want to extend the ride? We're all on a journey to live for as long as possible, enjoying the best quality of life we can, so if there's any chance of living longer I'm definitely taking it.

One of the ways to live longer is to reduce any bad habits and make healthier choices. Ultimately, we are a product of our actions and our habits, and due to stressful and busy lifestyles, it's very easy to form habits that give us a short-term buzz, high or release, but in the long term can be very detrimental to our health. Below are some of the most common habits that have a detrimental effect on your health, but the good news is that many of them are easily reversible and I see people make changes all the time to successfully cut them out, so I'm confident that you can too!

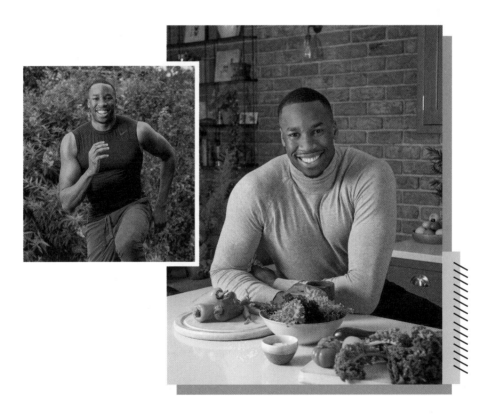

Why we should all quit smoking

Everyone knows how common smoking is – there are 1.4 million smokers in the UK alone! And although the UK government has introduced a number of different ways to try to cut down smoking, especially in public areas, unfortunately it is still a huge problem. According to Cancer Research UK, smoking is the biggest single preventable cause of illness and early death. Every year almost 78,000 people in the UK will die from smoking and many of us have smoking-related chronic conditions. Smoking is one of the biggest modifiable risk factors for cancer: of the mouth, throat, lungs, cervix, liver, stomach… the list goes on. Not only that, it is one of the biggest risks for developing long-term heart disease, vascular disease and stroke. A lot of these conditions, although treatable, are irreversible, which shows just how dangerous smoking can be.

We also know that smoking increases the chance of developing many chronic respiratory lung diseases such as emphysema, fibrotic lung disease and lung cancer. Smoking also increases the chances of being more unwell from acute diseases such as Covid-19. Covid-19 is a disease caused by a respiratory virus, and people who smoke generally have an increased risk of contracting any respiratory illness – and you're more likely to get severe symptoms if you are a smoker. We know that smoking causes damage to the lungs and airways and weakens the immune system, and ultimately reduces the body's ability to fight infection. We also know that smoking is bad for the cardiovascular system and can affect the blood vessels in the body and around the heart. This is going to weaken the body overall and makes it harder to fight disease.

And the thing about smoking is that it doesn't just affect you – it affects everybody around you. Passive smoking also increases the chances of developing long-term chronic health conditions related to smoking.

Stopping smoking can help to bring immediate benefits to your long-term health and your cardiovascular system. After quitting smoking, your oxygen levels recover within just a few hours and you'll find it easier to breathe after 72 hours.

After 2–12 weeks your blood circulation will improve, and after quitting smoking for just one year your chances of developing heart disease halves compared to a smoker, with the risk of death from lung cancer also halving after ten years.

However, I do understand that, when it comes to quitting smoking, it's easier said than done. Therefore, if you smoke, it's important that you seek out support. There are many support methods available to help you stop smoking and getting the right help increases the chances of you stopping by three times and also reduces the chance of relapse once you've stopped. A number of different options exist, such as prescription tablets and nicotine replacement therapy, or even e-cigarettes. You can always get expert advice from your local smoking cessation service or GP. Make sure to download the free NHS Quit Smoking app to find out more.

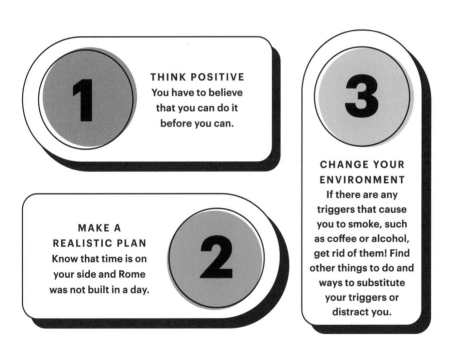

1 THINK POSITIVE
You have to believe that you can do it before you can.

2 MAKE A REALISTIC PLAN
Know that time is on your side and Rome was not built in a day.

3 CHANGE YOUR ENVIRONMENT
If there are any triggers that cause you to smoke, such as coffee or alcohol, get rid of them! Find other things to do and ways to substitute your triggers or distract you.

Stay away from too much alcohol

Alcohol, when taken responsibly, can be a genuinely refreshing beverage. However, regularly drinking more than 14 units of alcohol a week risks damaging your health.

WHAT 14 UNITS OF ALCOHOL LOOKS LIKE:

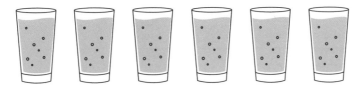

6 pints of beer *(4% strength)*

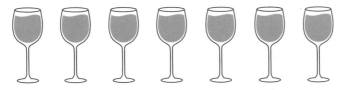

7 glasses of wine *(11.5% strength, 175ml)*

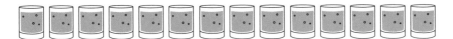

14 single shots of spirits *(40% strength)*

There is a lot of research about the effects of long-term drinking being related to chronic illnesses such as cancer. Regularly drinking more than 14 units a week for 10–20 years can increase your risk of cancers of the mouth and throat, stroke, heart disease, liver disease and even brain damage. Binge drinking and drinking too much in a single session can result in accidents and injury, and sometimes death, misjudging risky situations, losing self-control and engaging in risky behaviours such as violence and unprotected sex. It was once thought that some level of alcohol was good for the heart, but this has since been revised. If you're drinking fewer than 14 units a week this is still considered adequate or moderate drinking rather than safe because there is no 'safe' drinking level.

We know all about the physiological effects of alcohol; however, we need to be more aware of the effects of heavy drinking on mental health too, which can be just as bad or even worse. Alcohol affects the part of the brain which is associated with inhibition and therefore in the short term can make you feel more confident, less anxious and more relaxed. However, regular heavy drinking can actually make you feel worse in the long run, force you to drink more regularly and leave you feeling more anxious and depressed.

Alcohol has an effect on the chemicals and processes in the brain. It is also a depressant which disrupts the balance and affects your mood, your thoughts, your feelings and your actions. Experts are sure that those who have been depressed and drinking, when they are eventually able to stop and find other stress-free ways to relax, in time start to feel much better.

SIGNS THAT DRINKING MAY BE HAVING A NEGATIVE EFFECT ON YOUR HEALTH INCLUDE:

- **you find it hard to sleep**
- **you feel tired and hungover regularly**
- **you are unnecessarily anxious and worried in places and circumstances you wouldn't normally be**
- **you find it harder to maintain healthy relationships**

Try to resist the urge to reach for the bottle any time you feel anxious or down and see if you can break the habit. Start by cutting down, keeping a drink diary as well as having smaller, weaker drinks. Also make sure you incorporate drink-free days into your week. To relax and unwind in other more healthy ways, try doing some exercise, yoga, stretching, listening to calm music, having a relaxing bath or simply hanging out with friends. When you feel confident enough, you can even try a month without alcohol such as 'Dry January'.

It's important to regulate your consumption of alcohol, and these simple health hacks can support you in trying to cut down:

- **Have regular breaks from drinking and have alcohol-free days.**
- **Drink alcohol-free alternatives.**
- **Stay hydrated, drinking water between alcoholic drinks.**
- **Set a budget on what you're going to spend on alcohol before you go out.**
- **Swap stronger drinks for weaker drinks – lay off the spirits where possible!**
- **Let family and friends know you are trying to cut down so they are aware and can support you, but also hold you accountable.**

By cutting down on your drinking you can feel better and fresher in the mornings and less tired during the day – and your long-term health will reap the benefits too.

BENEFITS OF CUTTING DOWN ON DRINKING

Reducing your drinking will help you to:

- **avoid symptoms like headaches and confusion**
- **improve your mood, sleep and your immune system**
- **be more energetic**
- **improve the appearance of your skin and have better general long-term health**

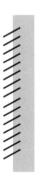

Medical myth

'HAIR OF THE DOG' CURES HANGOVERS

The hair-of-the-dog approach, which involves drinking more alcohol to relieve the hangover, doesn't actually help. I suggest, just don't do it. Trust me on this one – it's not worth it and may only make symptoms worse.

How long does alcohol stay in your system?

On average, we tend to metabolise about half a drink per hour for the average size person. But so many factors play a part in this, such as your age, your size, what you've had to drink, how many units are in your drink and how much you have eaten.

It's noted that even if your body can clear alcohol from the bloodstream at an average rate of 1 unit per hour, a breathalyser and blood test can still detect alcohol for up to 12 hours. And a urine test can detect it for up to 3–5 days, while a hair test can detect it for up to 90 days. So if you're going to be driving or operating heavy machinery, it's best you just don't drink at all. Even if this means you're not as merry or fun as you would like to be at that party or on a date... And if you're not sure whether you can drive the morning after, don't take the risk and just don't drive. Trying to predict your alcohol clearance exactly is harder than trying to predict the British weather!

THAT DREADED HANGOVER

We know that too much of anything can be a bad thing, but this is especially apparent when it comes to alcohol. We've already discussed the serious effects of alcohol, both in the short- and long-term, but many of us have still had far too much on a night out and suffered the effects of that deadly hangover the next morning. Symptoms include:

- **excessive thirst**
- **headache**
- **body aches**
- **fatigue**
- **anxiety and low mood**
- **dizziness**
- **nausea and vomiting**
- **trembling**

The severity of a hangover is closely related to factors such as how much alcohol you've consumed, how much sleep you've had, hydration levels, the pacing of alcoholic drinks and how many different drinks you had. Although back in 2017 I did do a fun video with the BBC about hangover cures, there isn't actually a cure as such, but rather ways in which you can reduce the symptoms and aid recovery. These include:

- **drinking water: alcohol often makes us pee a lot and leads to dehydration – it's therefore critical to rehydrate the body**
- **eating nutritious and healthy foods containing good antioxidants**
- **eating some fruit: the fructose in the fruit may help the body break down that alcohol**
- **getting plenty of rest and sleep**

Sometimes headache symptoms can be relieved with over-the-counter medication, such as pain-relief medication, but be careful because certain medications which affect the liver can make the symptoms worse, so if you have any health issues make sure you seek medical advice. And if you're suffering from a hangover over and over again, it might be worth getting some support to help you cut down on drinking to aid your long-term health and well-being.

A good way to prevent a hangover is to avoid alcohol entirely. But, let's be honest, if you're out you may not want to do that, so make sure to drink in moderation, giving plenty of time for your body to process the alcohol before consuming more. It's also worth bearing in mind that each person's tolerance is different.

WHAT MEDICATIONS SHOULD I NOT TAKE WITH ALCOHOL?

Many people are aware that when taking medication we have to be careful of what else we are taking – and alcohol is one of those substances that can either inhibit or amplify the effects of medication in an uncontrolled and unpredictable way.

- **A simple cold pill that makes you drowsy can make you unconscious if taken with too much alcohol. We advise you to avoid alcohol while taking allergy and cold medication.**

- **We advise not to drink alcohol while taking medicines for angina which can lower blood pressure and cause abnormal heart rhythms.**

- **There are drugs that can be used to help relieve anxiety and panic attacks that can cause life-threatening symptoms if taken with enough alcohol. And note that there are some non-steroidal anti-inflammatory drugs (NSAIDs), such as high-strength ibuprofen or naproxen, which can cause severe side effects such as ulcers and stomach bleeding, especially in older people, when taken with alcohol.**

- **It's advisable to avoid alcohol while taking a course of antibiotics. However, if drinking in moderation and sensibly it's unlikely there will be any permanent damage caused by drinking while taking antibiotics. There are certain antibiotics, however, that we advise definitely not to drink with: one is metronidazole, which is an antibiotic used for vaginal, dental and sometimes abdominal infections. You might have symptoms such as vomiting, abdominal pain, nausea, headaches, dizziness or drowsiness. Always check the information leaflet and speak to your doctor before drinking while taking antibiotics.**

- **Certain medications like doxycycline, used to treat sexually transmitted infections (STIs) and chest infections, may not work as well if you have chronic liver problems from alcohol.**

If you have any concerns or queries and feel that your medication course might be affected by alcohol, you should speak to your GP or pharmacist as they can provide more specific information, depending on the medication you're taking and how long you've been taking it for.

The drugs just don't work

Recent studies have shown that substance abuse has been linked to developing a number of chronic diseases related to various organs. Substance abusers are more likely to be hospitalised from a simple infection as they're more prone to a weakened immune system. The lungs and cardiovascular system are often compromised and that may explain why they get so ill if they get Covid-19 or other acute bacterial, fungal and viral illnesses.

There are also many ways that drugs can impact your mental health. Drugs can affect your mood, mind and behaviour, and have been linked to chronic conditions such as depression, anxiety and schizophrenia. Regular use of drugs means people can become dependent on them and this can have a negative impact on day-to-day life, such as problems with money, education and employment, relationships, housing, low self-esteem and finding it hard to maintain commitments. Substance abuse can also lead to crime, violence and even imprisonment.

One of the issues with taking drugs is that you don't always know what's in them and it can be difficult to predict how your body may react. They could include additional harmful substances and may not even contain any of the substance you're expecting to take. Even if you've taken something before, drugs can contain different ingredients when taken the next time. This is more likely to be the case with illegal highs, such as illegal market opiates like heroin, stimulants like cocaine, certain depressants and also psychoactive drugs such as ecstasy.

Roughly 50 per cent of individuals with severe mental disorders are affected by substance abuse, and 37 per cent of alcohol abusers and 50 per cent of drug abusers also have at least one serious mental illness. Of all the people diagnosed with mental illness, 29 per cent abuse alcohol or drugs, and if you have an existing mental health condition, drug abuse can make it so much worse.

We all know that drug abuse can be life-ruining and life-threatening. But it doesn't just affect you – it can affect everyone around you, such as friends, family, co-workers and loved ones. It's important that if you, or someone close to you, are suffering from drug addiction, you seek help immediately. The NHS and GP services offer a number of different ways to treat drug abuse depending on what drug you're addicted to and how long you've been addicted. Please don't be afraid to reach out.

A&E STORY

I was asked to see a 24-year-old gentleman who came in to A&E with extreme abdominal pain. He said he had tried many different over-the-counter painkillers and medication; however, the pain was just getting worse.

I took a full history of the signs and symptoms and wondered to myself what was causing the pain and which investigations I would choose to do. He said that he had previously been quite fit and well and didn't have any family medical problems. The only particular thing I'd noted in his history was that he said he had been to a very wild party a few days before coming to hospital.

After a number of blood tests and scans, we found out he had cocaine-induced intestinal ischaemia. This is a very rare condition where cocaine abuse causes a disruption in the blood supply to the gut causing pain and bowel abnormalities. The man spoke to me about his drug history and said that he often takes the occasional recreational drug at large parties. After treating him, I spoke to him about how sometimes social behaviour can affect your health. A number of young people who feel that they may be invincible to health scares and medical problems often play Russian roulette with their health by taking a number of different, dangerous drugs at parties. I let him know how cocaine works and the physiological effects it can have on your body. I hope that the scare of what happened and what he went through, along with the advice I gave him, will support him to change his health behaviours for the better and hopefully he can pass on that knowledge to others.

OTHER REGULAR HABITS

that could be harming our health

There are a number of habits many of us do knowingly and unknowingly that may be harming our health in the long term:

1

SLOUCHING

This is something that many of us do and the results bring people swarming into GP practices across the country with chronic lower back pain. With people sitting at their computers for many hours every day, this is fast becoming one of the biggest issues GPs see. So fix up, look sharp, shoulders back and sit up tall!

2

INCREASED USE OF SOCIAL MEDIA AND DEVICES

There have been a number of studies showing that an increased use of social media and devices is linked to worrying, anxiety, depression and poor sleep. Social media can be a great place for positive change – and I have experienced this through my work with TikTok. However, it's good to switch off, build healthy boundaries and make sure you make good personal connections in real life and have some down time from screen time. See pages 185–6 for more on this.

3

FAILING TO CHANGE YOUR BEDSHEETS

A lot of us sleep with the same bedsheets for an extended amount of time, which can increase the risk of skin disease, bacteria and bedbugs. We should be changing our bedding weekly.

4

KNUCKLE-CRACKING

All the rumours say that cracking your knuckles can cause arthritis in the long term, though there are no official studies proving that. However, we do know that extended knuckle-cracking, which is the popping of the nitrogen in the synovial fluid of the joints, can lead to weakening of the joints, so it's probably best avoided.

5

SLEEP DEPRIVATION

Lack of sleep is known to be linked to a number of different diseases, can prevent people being able to function properly on a day-to-day basis and can also cause poor sex drive, poor concentration, irritability, stress, reduced energy, mood changes, lack of energy and regular headaches, which is another very common presentation we see in GP practices and in A&E. See pages 172–3 for some tips on getting a good night's sleep.

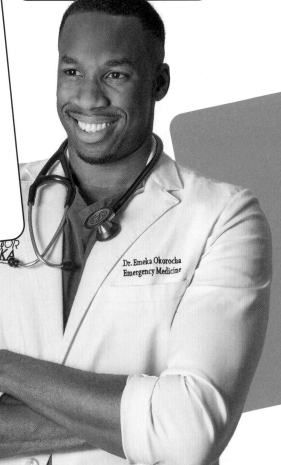

Dr. Emeka Okorocha
Emergency Medicine

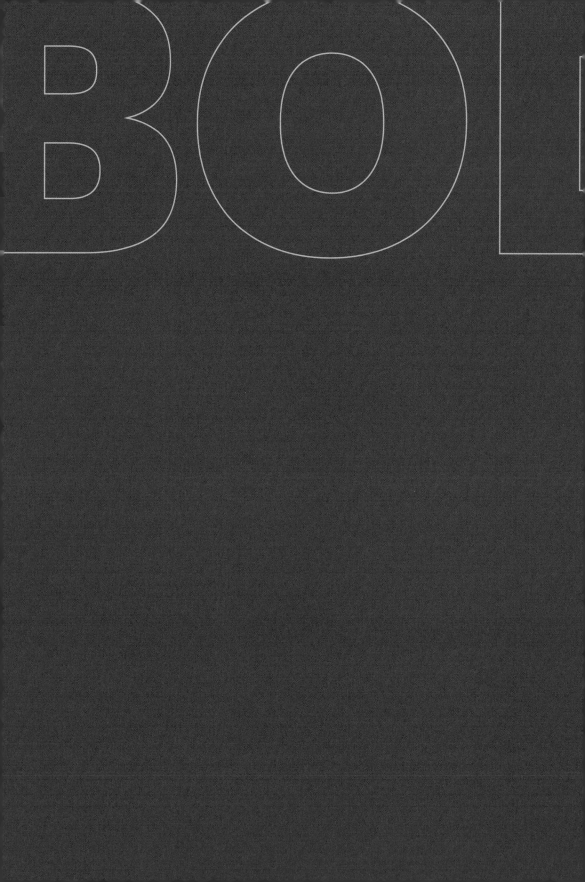

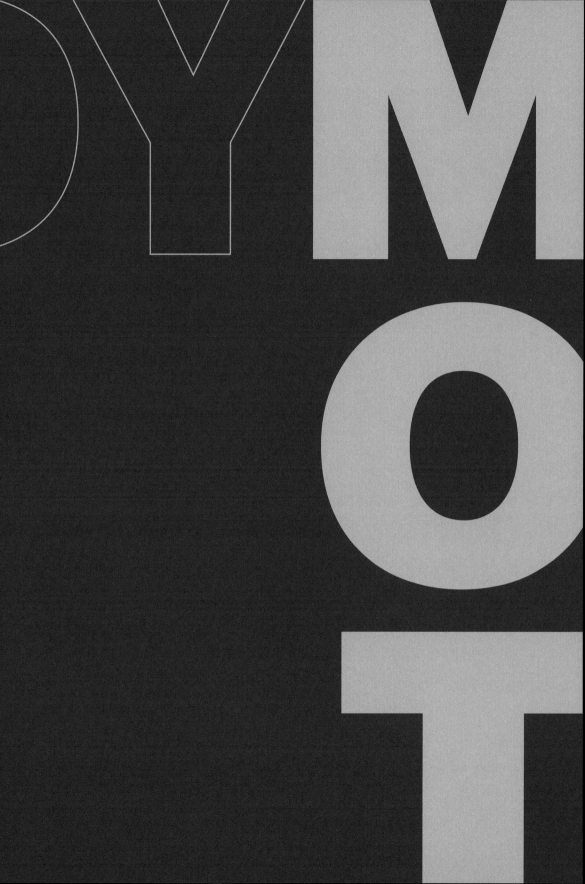

GETTING YOUR BODY IN ORDER

MOTIVATION

Too many of us don't see Monday for what it truly is – an opportunity, a chance, a blessing. Unfortunately, in my job I've seen so many people who won't get to experience another Monday. So next time you find yourself dreading Monday or you take it as just another day, think, 'This is a blessing I get to experience that so many others can't, and I'm going to make the very best of it!'

The gravity of what can happen when we don't take care of ourselves both mentally and physically is indisputable, and as a frontline doctor who has seen first-hand the devastating effects of disease, I feel it's my moral and ethical responsibility to use the knowledge I've gained, both professionally and personally, to give you the tools to make your health a priority and, by doing so, not only hopefully prolong, but also improve the quality of, your life.

I mean, you only have one body, so why not make it the best you can? They say your body is a temple for a reason. So you need to keep your temple in the best condition possible. If you could look into the future and see how your negative body habits could cause you significant harm later in life, you'd want to go back in time to make the right changes to get the best results. So now is the time to do it, and now you have this book to help you.

WHERE ARE YOU AT?

Before we dive in, let's check in with how you are feeling health-wise:

- **Are you happy with your current health?**
- **Do you ever find yourself overly tired?**
- **How much sleep do you get at night?**
- **Do you feel you could be healthier?**
- **Do you suffer from a long-term health condition?**
- **Does your current weight fit within recommended guidelines?**
- **Do you smoke at all? If so, how much?**
- **Do you drink alcohol? If so, are you within the recommended limits?**
- **How often do you need to visit the doctor with persistent symptoms?**
- **How do you keep track of your health?**

There are also some basic, but important, things you should be doing every day:

- **Have you moved your body?**
- **Have you drunk enough water?**
- **Have you got your daily intake of fruit and veg?**
- **Have you taken a few mindful minutes?**
- **Have you laughed today?**

In this chapter we will explore both the serious and sinister health issues, such as cancer and heart disease, as well as those day-to-day issues that aren't as life-threatening but still affect us nonetheless, such as hair loss and urinary tract infections.

Heart disease

The heart is a major muscle in the body about the size of a fist, and it pumps blood around your body about 70 times a minute. The heart has its own blood supply from vessels on the surface called the coronary arteries. When these get blocked this can lead to heart attack. Coronary heart disease is one of the major causes of death in the UK and worldwide. It is sometimes called ischaemic heart disease or coronary artery disease.

HOW TO RECOGNISE IF YOU ARE HAVING A HEART ATTACK

- chest pain or pain elsewhere in the body, often the arms, neck, jaw, stomach or back
- shortness of breath, wheezing or coughing
- feeling faint or dizzy
- feeling or being sick
- an overwhelming sense of unease

If you have any of these symptoms, seek urgent medical advice.

It's important to know that not everyone has the same symptoms and you may not have any symptoms before you are diagnosed with coronary heart disease. Causes are from a process called atherosclerosis where fatty deposits are distributed around the vessels. This can be prevented by improving lifestyle factors, such as stopping smoking, reducing drinking and taking regular exercise. Therefore, we tend to recommend lifestyle changes as our first choice of treatment, though we can then go on to prescribing medication and sometimes even carrying out an angioplasty – where balloons or stents are used to treat narrow vessels.

A&E STORY

One time in the emergency department I saw a 67-year-old lady who came in presenting with chest pain and difficulty breathing. She had a history of chest pain and had sought medical care a few years previously and was diagnosed with a heart attack. Unfortunately, she had risk factors, such as hypertension (high blood pressure) and type 2 diabetes, and she was a long-term smoker.

Once we treated her in A&E for the chest pain we did a number of different investigations which showed that her blood vessels, which provide the heart with oxygen, were very narrow. This led to her having heart failure and chronic ischaemic heart disease. We were able to clinically treat her for her symptoms in A&E by starting her on some medications to reduce her blood pressure, keep her diabetes in check and to try to dilate some of her blood vessels. We also counselled her about her diet and lifestyle choices such as smoking. We had to clearly explain to her that even with the intervention of medications, if she didn't change her lifestyle choices, there was a chance she wouldn't live very long. We gave her all the medical help and advice we could and referred her to a specialist.

How to lower your cholesterol

We know how serious cholesterol is as a factor in developing heart and vessel disease.

THE MAIN WAYS OF LOWERING YOUR CHOLESTEROL INCLUDE:

- cutting out saturated fats and trans fats, and increasing the amount of omega-3 fatty acids and fibre you eat
- physical activity
- losing weight
- stopping smoking
- limiting alcohol intake

Medical myth

ALL CHOLESTEROL IS BAD FOR YOU

A lot of cholesterol may be bad for you, but not all cholesterol is. We need some cholesterol, and the good cholesterol is known as high-density lipoprotein (HDL), which helps the body make hormones, cell membranes and vitamin D. Low-density lipoprotein (LDL) tends to be the 'bad' cholesterol which clogs the arteries. The balance of the two is what determines how healthy you are, rather than how much cholesterol is actually there.

Hypertension (aka high blood pressure)

Hypertension is a huge preventable issue, especially in the western world. It is estimated that over 1.5 billion people worldwide have high blood pressure and it has been linked to some of the most serious diseases, such as ischaemic heart disease, cancer, diabetes, stroke and myocardial infarction, aka heart attacks.

THE BEST WAY TO REDUCE YOUR BLOOD PRESSURE IS NATURALLY BY ADDRESSING CERTAIN LIFESTYLE FACTORS:

- **maintaining a healthy weight**
- **reducing your salt intake**
- **increasing your daily physical activity**
- **stopping smoking and limiting alcohol consumption**
- **reducing stress and anxiety**
- **getting a good night's sleep**

There are also some aspects that we can't control, such as our genetics, our race and our gender, which all play a part. When lifestyle modification factors don't work, there are a number of different treatment options for high blood pressure, but most of the time it can be controlled by you!

How to recognise the signs of a stroke

F: if you see facial droop on any side;
A: if there's any new weakness in either arm;
S: if there is any kind of irregular new speech issue;
T: time to call 999.

When it comes to strokes, time is one of the most important factors. In the emergency department, we have a specific window of time from the onset of symptoms to the diagnosis, which affects treatment. So if you think you or somebody else is having a stroke, get medical attention immediately.

Diabetes

There are different types of diabetes, but the one we most talk about is due to a lack of, or resistance to, insulin, a natural hormone that reduces your blood sugar. It's important to differentiate between type 1 and type 2. Type 1 diabetics are usually diagnosed when they are younger, and suffer from a disorder where the body destroys the cells that make insulin. Type 2 diabetics generally develop a resistance to their body's insulin in later life.

According to the World Health Organization (WHO), about 422 million people worldwide have diabetes – and more than 95 per cent of people with diabetes have type 2, which many doctors feel can be preventable.

LET'S WORK TOGETHER TO GET DIABETES UNDER CONTROL

Risk factors that can be controlled include:

- **improving diet**
- **increasing exercise**
- **reducing obesity**

A&E STORY

A 41-year-old woman came in to A&E with a history of dizziness, and feeling unusually light-headed. She said she'd been having symptoms for the last three days and she didn't understand why. She wasn't taking any medications, nor did she smoke or drink. She claimed she tried to keep healthy and was doing vigorous exercise every day. Her examination findings were generally unremarkable.

It was very difficult for me to diagnose her initially. We did a number of investigations, such as blood and urine tests and we checked her blood sugars. It was after doing the latter that we realised what the problem was. Although her diet had been normal and she'd been genuinely very fit and healthy, she didn't realise that because she had a strong family history of diabetes, she could have medical problems too.

We referred her to the diabetic team who were able to correct her blood sugars and the symptoms were resolved. I explained to her the importance of having health checks at least once a year even if you don't have symptoms. The genuine misconception is that if you live a healthy life you're immune to any disease, but that's not always the case. I advise people to live a healthy life and drink responsibly, but to also make sure that they're checking on their health regularly and that they have a good idea of their family health history. We advise if you're healthy and not taking regular medication or dealing with chronic disease, you should aim to see your doctor every five years if aged 40–74, though this will vary from person to person.

Cancer

Many cancers, such as breast and ovarian cancer, have genetic links. However, there are a number of modifiable risk factors such as obesity, diet, smoking, alcohol and lifestyle tendencies – like using sunbeds or having unprotected sexual intercourse – which increase the chances of some cancers developing. In the UK the most common cancers are breast, bowel, prostate and lung.

If more than one family member on the same side has the same type of cancer or they develop the cancer before the age of 50 this puts you at greater risk. If you have any worries about developing a certain cancer, or you recognise any of the following signs and symptoms, it's advisable to speak to your GP because a number of tests can be run to ensure anything identified is done so early.

BREAST CANCER

Breast cancer is the most common cancer in the UK – around 55,000 women and 370 men are diagnosed each year – and it is one of the most common causes of death from cancer. It is much more common in women than in men and is a leading cause of death in women under 50.

Risk factors include:

- age
- family history
- a previous history of breast cancer
- not having had a child or breastfed a child
- early puberty or late menopause
- hormone replacement therapy (HRT) in menopause
- long-term use of the combined contraceptive pill can have a small increased risk

SIGNS AND SYMPTOMS OF BREAST CANCER

- breast pain
- a new breast lump (often painless)
- nipple changes or discharge
- a change in the size or shape of one or both breasts
- skin contour changes, such as dimpling, puckering or redness
- a lump or swelling in either armpit

How should I check my breasts?

There is not necessarily a right or wrong way to check your breasts, but it is so important to check them regularly so you can notice any changes. Just as body shapes differ in terms of appearance and size, so too do breasts and it's perfectly normal for one breast to be longer or larger than the other. What's important is that you know what's normal for you, to look at them and feel them regularly, know what changes to look out for and, if you see any, speak to your GP without delay. You should also attend your routine screening if you're aged 50–71.

Look out for changes in the size, outline or shape of your breasts, or the look and feel of the skin on your breasts such as a rash or redness. Any new lump, swelling or thickening of the breast area should be checked out or if there is noticeable discharge or fluid from either of your nipples, see your GP straight away. If there's any change in the position or any severe discomfort or pain in one of the breasts, especially if there is a new pain that doesn't go away and isn't cyclical, you should inform your GP.

BOWEL CANCER

Bowel cancer is the fourth most common cancer in the UK and is the second most common cause of cancer death. Each year nearly 6 in 10 new cases are diagnosed in people aged 70 and over, but it can affect people of any age. The most common site for bowel cancer is the rectum.

Risk factors include:
- **a positive family history**
- **a diet rich in meat and fat, and poor in fibre**
- **inflammatory bowel disease**
- **race (it is more common in Caucasian people than Black and Asian people)**
- **high alcohol intake**
- **smoking**
- **a sedentary lifestyle**
- **obesity**

SIGNS AND SYMPTOMS OF BOWEL CANCER

- **weight loss**
- **abdominal pain or discomfort**
- **rectal bleeding**
- **a change in bowel habit**
- **blood in the stool**
- **anaemia**

PROSTATE CANCER

Prostate cancer is the most common cancer in men and makes up 27 per cent of all UK cancers. It affects 1 in 8 men in the UK at some point in their lives, with a high incidence in males aged 75–79.

Risk factors include:
- **increasing age**
- **race (it is more common in Black men than Caucasian or Asian men)**
- **obesity**
- **a positive family history**
- **poor food and alcohol consumption**

SIGNS AND SYMPTOMS OF PROSTATE CANCER

Prostate cancer doesn't often cause symptoms. However, if you do have symptoms, they might include:

- **loss of appetite (anorexia)**
- **weight loss**
- **bone pain**
- **an enlarged prostate**
- **urinary frequency or changes**
- **blood in the pee or semen**
- **impotence**
- **suprapubic pain**

LUNG CANCER

There are approximately 48,000 new cases of lung cancer diagnosed in the UK every year. Almost 90 per cent of lung cancers are caused by smoking and it is the biggest cause of death from cancer in the UK. 53 per cent of lung cancer diagnoses are in males, and 47 per cent in females.

Risk factors include:

- **active or passive smoking**
- **increasing age**
- **history of other cancer and chronic lung disease**
- **industrial dust diseases or exposure to asbestos or radiation**
- **family history of lung disease and lung cancer**

SIGNS AND SYMPTOMS OF LUNG CANCER

- **coughing up blood**
- **a persistent cough**
- **recurrent chest infections**
- **breathlessness**
- **weight loss or loss of appetite**
- **bone pain**
- **tiredness and lethargy**
- **chronic wheeze and stridor (noisy breathing)**
- **voice hoarseness**
- **chest or shoulder pain**

Do you have asthma?

Asthma is a reversible obstruction of the airways. It's an inflammatory condition, but it's also a condition of hyper responsiveness which can be triggered by a number of factors, such as dust, pets and allergies, outdoor pollution, mould, tobacco smoke or viral infections. Acute severe asthma could be life-threatening and chronic asthma can cause significant problems to people's lives. Most chronic asthma cases are treated in primary care by the GP; however, acute asthma attacks are treated by doctors like myself in the emergency department and require immediate medical attention.

Asthma is a very common, yet very deadly, disease: 5.4 million people in the UK are currently being treated for asthma and it affects 1 in 11 children and approximately 1 in 12 adults. Asthma is actually the most prevalent chronic medical condition in children, though many grow out of childhood asthma when treated accordingly. Asthma more commonly occurs in women than men, which can possibly be explained physiologically by the changing hormone levels in the menstrual cycle. Pregnancy and menopause can also make asthma symptoms worse. Women's lungs are also smaller than men's, which means that they're more sensitive to asthma triggers and it makes it harder for women to breathe when they're having an asthma attack.

> **Every 10 seconds someone in the UK has a potentially life-threatening asthma attack. So please, if you're asthmatic, make sure you always have your inhaler with you and if you get breathless and it's not relieved by 10 puffs of your inhaler, call the emergency services immediately. Signs of an asthma attack include getting chesty, wheezy and struggling to breathe.**

Why should we see the GP regularly?

You should be seeing your GP regularly, especially if you are taking medication. This is because medication needs to be reviewed and evaluated. Seeing a GP and having a physical examination and your history taken can also identify chronic, deadly illnesses before they progress and get serious. The earlier we find illnesses such as cancer, the better treatment outcome you have. It's also useful to see your GP regularly so you are informed about your health such as the screening tests you're eligible for.

Often when people come to see us in A&E, there are underlying issues or illnesses that have been worrying them that they have ignored and left untreated. It can be really overwhelming to bite the bullet and see your doctor – to make that appointment – especially if you are fearful, but if you notice anything unusual at all, see your GP as soon as you can to give you peace of mind or get the help you need.

Obesity

Our risk of having poor health or developing more serious diseases rises substantially as body mass index (BMI) increases. We use BMI as a measurement for obesity. If your BMI is over 30 this means you're obese and if it's over 40 it means you're severely obese. Sometimes this isn't an accurate reading because BMI can be very high for someone who is very muscular but doesn't have much fat. And so sometimes we will measure waist size as well.

Living with excess weight puts people at a greater risk from any disease. Figures show that one of the biggest risk factors for becoming seriously ill with chronic disease is obesity. In general in the UK over 11,000 hospital admissions a year can be attributable to obesity, and the majority of adults in the UK are overweight or obese – 67 per cent of men and 60 per cent of women – and therefore at greater risk of acute and chronic disease. It's estimated that being obese or overweight contributes to at least 1 in every 13 deaths in Europe. And being obese can reduce life expectancy from 3 to 20 years depending on the severity. These numbers show just how important it is to have your weight under control.

OBESITY CAUSES MANY PROBLEMS AND SERIOUS HEALTH CONDITIONS.

Day-to-day problems people with obesity may face include:

- breathlessness
- increased sweating
- snoring + disrupted sleep
- difficulty doing simple activities
- joint + back pain
- low self-esteem
- feeling isolated
- fertility issues

More chronic serious conditions could include:

- asthma
- high blood pressure
- heart disease
- some cancers
- osteoarthritis
- liver disease
- kidney disease
- diabetes
- issues in pregnancy

The best way to treat obesity is eating a balanced diet (see pages 94–119) and natural weight-loss management, or joining a local weight-loss group and making sure to exercise daily (see pages 152–70).

A&E STORY

I saw an overweight 50-year-old gentleman in A&E. He had seen his GP many times because he kept falling asleep – it was getting worse and they hadn't been able to find a cause. It had become so bad that he had fallen asleep doing an activity and banged his head. I treated him for his head wounds which were not serious, but the aim was to discover why he was so tired all the time.

We performed the usual investigations and took a clear history and examination. However, we still couldn't find a conclusive cause for his excessive sleepiness. I believed that, due to his excessive weight, it could be being caused by obstructive sleep apnoea (OSA), but only certain tests would be able to prove this. OSA is a condition that occurs when the walls of the throat relax and narrow while you sleep, which means your breathing stops and starts. I referred the man for some tests for further investigation and told him to come back any time if he continued to have issues.

A few weeks later, I met him again – this time with his child who I was coincidentally treating in paediatric A&E. He told me that after having the tests I had referred him for, along with taking part in some sleep studies, the GP confirmed that he had indeed got OSA. One of the major causes of OSA is being overweight. I discussed this with him and he said the GP had also told him that his BMI and neck size were probably contributory factors. I chatted to him about different ways he could lose weight which would help him have better sleep patterns and I explained how being overweight could harm his health in other ways too.

It was a fulfilling moment because I was able to use my knowledge of lifestyle habits as an indicator of what I believed he was suffering from. Sometimes in A&E we see cases that don't go the way we want them to, but it is so rewarding when they do and it's a great feeling when our help can change people's lives for the better.

Facts about obesity

2

THE PROBLEM WITH OBESITY

Obesity is such a common problem in the UK and it's estimated to affect around 1 in 4 adults and 1 in 5 children aged 10–11.

1

OBESITY & DISEASE

Obesity is so important to tackle because, as well as physical changes, it can lead to a number of severely life-threatening conditions, such as diabetes, heart disease and some types of cancer.

4

OBESITY & DIET

There are many medical causes for obesity, such as metabolic and hormonal disorders and thyroid issues. However, when it comes to lifestyle, obesity comes down to consuming a lot more calories, particularly from fatty and sugary foods, than you're burning. And then the excess energy is stored in the body as fat.

3

THE TERM 'OBESE'

The term 'obese' refers to somebody who is very overweight with a lot of body fat.

How can I stop snoring?

If you're overweight, start by tackling that first and shedding the pounds. Then you can try some of the following:

- Try changing the way you sleep: sleep on your side not your back.
- Use extra pillows or raise your head up to help open your airways.
- Treat any nasal congestion or obstructions.
- Limit drinking alcohol and taking sedatives before bed.
- Reduce or ideally stop smoking.
- Use nasal strips or an external nasal dilator.
- Make sure you're getting enough and regular sleep.

Urinary tract infections (UTIs)

UTIs are infections that affect the urinary tract, such as cystitis (which affects the bladder), urethritis (which affects the urethra) or pyelonephritis (which affects the kidneys). Women are 14 times more likely to get UTIs than men.

SYMPTOMS INCLUDE:

- **burning and pain when you pee**
- **needing to pee more frequently**
- **your pee appearing cloudy**
- **blood in your pee**
- **pain in the abdomen and in the back or just under the ribs**

For really bad infections, symptoms can include a high temperature, feeling feverish, hot and shivery, or a very low temperature. At this point you need to seek urgent medical advice.

Eight ways to prevent UTIs

1 AVOID SUGARY FOODS AND DRINKS

2 KEEP THE GENITAL AREA CLEAN AND DRY AND CHANGE UNDERWEAR

3 AVOID HOLDING IN YOUR PEE WHEN YOU HAVE THE URGE TO GO

REGULARLY WASH THE GENITALS **4**

5 DRINK PLENTY OF FLUIDS – MAINLY WATER

6 MAKE SURE TO PEE AFTER ANY SEXTRACURRICULAR ACTIVITY

AVOID TIGHT, SYNTHETIC UNDERWEAR **7**

WIPE FROM FRONT TO BACK AFTER USING THE TOILET, ESPECIALLY FOR FEMALES **8**

Seasonal affective disorder (SAD)

SAD is a mood disorder in which people have good mental health throughout most of the year, but can exhibit depressive symptoms at the same time every year, normally in the winter. Often the change in weather and reduction in sunlight can be the cause. Common symptoms include lethargy, sleeping too much, having little energy and overeating. SAD affects about 3 in every 100 people in the UK. SAD is often classed as a unique mood disorder because it has a seasonal pattern. This can vary from having the winter blues and having feelings such as low mood and depression to feeling worthless and having thoughts of suicide. Sometimes it can result in withdrawal from activities and social interaction as well as poor sleep and loss of appetite. There is evidence that people who suffer from SAD have a change in their circadian rhythm (the body's internal clock). Management of symptoms includes things such as light therapy or even medication, such as antidepressants. Physical exercise is also used as an effective form of depression therapy which can help improve mood.

Hair loss

Most of the time, especially in males, hair loss is a natural process that occurs when we get older. Hair falls out as part of the body's natural renewal cycle. However, sometimes irregular hair loss can be caused by a condition, such as alopecia areata. This is an autoimmune condition – where the body's immune system attacks itself – and results in small patches of irregular baldness. Alopecia areata is not to be confused with alopecia totalis (when all the hair on your head is gone) or alopecia universalis (when all the hair on your body is gone). This affects men and women equally and often occurs before the age of 40. It is sometimes treated with steroid cream and, rest assured, the majority of the time the hair will grow back.

There are a few things we can do to avoid provocation of hair loss, such as:

- **avoiding hairstyles that are pulling at our hair**
- **avoiding high-heat hair-styling tools**
- **trying not to chemically bleach or use harsh shampoo on the hair**
- **using a soft rather than a hard brush**

If the condition persists, there are many medical options that your dermatologist can discuss with you.

CAN I GET A DOCTOR'S NOTE WITHOUT SEEING MY GP?

This is a really common question and there are a few factors that come into play here, such as why you're off sick, whether or not the GP needs to assess you face-to-face and whether or not you've been admitted to hospital. A sick note needs to be signed by a doctor, but you don't necessarily have to go and see your GP. If you contact the GP practice you may be able to get a consultation over the phone or they'll tell you if you need to come in and be seen. If you've been admitted to hospital, when you're being discharged the hospital doctor can write you a discharge letter. If you've seen another professional, the GP can use this as confirmation and write a sick note based on that.

As we've seen, small lifestyle changes, such as stopping smoking, maintaining a healthy weight, reducing stress and anxiety, getting a good night's sleep and increasing physical activity, really can make big, big differences to your future health. You will find advice on how to make these small modifications throughout this book.

Medical myth

SHAVING YOUR HAIR MAKES IT GROW BACK THICKER AND QUICKER

This is just a myth. Shaving doesn't affect the cells that cause your hair to grow back or the speed at which they do. Shaved hair may appear coarser but there is no difference in the actual thickness.

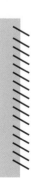

EMBARRASSING BODIES

MOTIVATION

Be happy with the body you've
been blessed with. Joy and
contentment on the inside
eventually manifest to beauty
on the outside, so make sure
to love the skin you're in!

Our bodies love to change and do weird and wonderful things. And these weird and wonderful things can sometimes be hugely embarrassing and leave us a tad bashful. Research shows that, when it comes to embarrassing conditions, almost two-thirds of patients would rather suffer in silence than seek help. But keeping your embarrassing problems on the down-low or a bit hush-hush can actually have a negative effect on your overall health in the long term. In this chapter we're going to talk about some of the most commonly seen embarrassing symptoms and conditions, and look at ways you can try to treat them at home, and identify when you need to seek medical help.

URINARY AND FAECAL INCONTINENCE

Having a little bit of a leak from the back passage – or anywhere else for that matter – can feel very embarrassing! However, incontinence – both urinary and faecal – can be caused by a number of different things, such as prostate, vaginal and rectal disorders, haemorrhoids, constipation, an overactive bladder, urinary infection and weakened pelvic muscles. Neurological disorders such as multiple sclerosis and even Alzheimer's disease can cause this too. So, how are we going to get rid of the old leak? Well, one thing you could try is Kegel exercises, which strengthen the pelvic floor muscles. A Kegel exercise is like pretending you need to pee or empty your bowels and then holding it in – clenching your muscles as if you were trying to stop it. You can do this throughout the day, squeezing for 10 seconds. This makes your muscles stronger and puts you more in control. Avoiding caffeinated and alcoholic drinks can also help with urinary incontinence and bulking up your fibre intake to 20–30g daily and avoiding caffeine, dairy, alcohol and sweeteners has been known to provide benefit for faecal incontinence.

BAD BREATH

Nobody wants to be known as 'yuck mouth', 'bin breath', 'hot tongue'... You get the point. So when it comes to bad breath you really want to do your best to get on top of it. There are certain medications which can cause you to have a dry mouth, which can cause bad breath. Alternatively, bad breath can be caused by foods containing sulphur, such as onions and garlic. However, it's mainly caused by bad dental hygiene, gum disease and cavities. Smoking and coffee don't help either. Try to avoid these substances, brush twice a day and scrub your tongue too. Using special toothpastes that contain sodium lauryl sulphate, along with brushing and flossing regularly, can help control oral bacteria, which can lead to bad breath. Drinking water and eating saliva-producing foods like apples and celery helps too.

PREMATURE EJACULATION

Sometimes, especially as we age, erections don't last long and climax comes a lot sooner than we'd like, and premature ejaculation is more common when coupled with erectile dysfunction (see opposite). When it comes to premature ejaculation, you can see that there are so many different causes. But many of us don't realise just how important the brain is when it comes to physical conditions such as premature ejaculation. Stress and what's on your mind often play a huge part. And it's good to note that many men have actually reported an improved sex life after combatting stress and getting their mental health in order.

Some of the causes of premature ejaculation include:

- **low amounts of the neurotransmitter serotonin**
- **stress**
- **guilt**
- **being overweight**
- **inflammation of the prostate or urethra**

There are a few things you can try to overcome premature ejaculation. Try to take a breather or a time out when you feel you're about to 'finish the job' or, if you're not trying to conceive, try using barrier contraception such as condoms to reduce sensitivity. Certain numbing creams can also help climax control. You could try Kegel exercises to strengthen your pelvic floor muscles (see page 67). If the cause is stress- or anxiety-related, it's not always about taking pills, such as antidepressants; sometimes talking therapy, behavioural therapy or incorporating stress-relieving techniques into your life – such as exercise, spending time with family members, going for walks or just having some downtime every now and then – can make a huge difference.

If you feel that premature ejaculation is really affecting your life and the methods I've mentioned haven't worked, have a chat with your GP and see what options are available to you.

ERECTILE DYSFUNCTION (IMPOTENCE)

This is embarrassing, I know, but it's important that we discuss it as it affects so many males globally, causing confidence and often relationship difficulties. Fifty per cent of British men in their thirties admit they've struggled in the bedroom and it's estimated that by 2025 more than 300 million men worldwide could be affected.

Risk factors include:

- **stress and anxiety**
- **tiredness**
- **obesity**
- **diabetes**
- **vascular problems**
- **cardiovascular disease**
- **high blood pressure**
- **drug use, smoking and alcohol**

If the problem persists, with no reversible cause, please seek medical attention!

VAGINAL ODOUR

The vagina is usually self-cleaning, but as beautiful as it can be, unfortunately sometimes it won't smell so sweet. This could be caused by a number of things, such as a sexually transmitted infection or disease, a yeast infection or just trapped moisture. Sometimes when you're going through the menopause the thinning of the vaginal lining can cause an unpleasant odour. Some of the things you can try to reduce vaginal odour are wearing cotton underwear and making sure you change your underwear daily and after you exercise. Try to avoid wearing tights and douching too.

If you think that you may have an infection and you have other symptoms, such as pain or discharge (see page 70), make sure to get checked or see a healthcare professional. Usually these can be treated with creams, suppositories or tablets. Sometimes eating an excess of food such as garlic, onions and asparagus can produce an odour, while having something sweet such as pineapples can help prevent it.

CAUSES OF VAGINAL DISCHARGE

- bacterial vaginosis
- sexual arousal
- yeast infection
- trichomoniasis (a sexually transmitted infection caused by a parasite)
- chlamydia and gonorrhoea
- pelvic inflammatory disease (PID)
- human papillomavirus (HPV)
- pregnancy
- birth control

BODY ODOUR

While we're on the topic of odours, sometimes your whole body can give off a bit of a whiff. Often when you have that funk your friends or people close to you will let you know – one way or another! However, if you notice it yourself, there are a few things you can do to try to prevent it. Make sure you wash at least once a day with soap and water and after exercise or any episode of excessive sweating. If you live with obesity or have excess fat, make sure you wash under the creases to make sure there is no bacteria or sweat left there.

EXCESSIVE SWEATING

Sweating is very natural and happens to many of us in many different situations. However, if you're always drenched like you've been out in British rain, it can make everyday tasks difficult and have a severe negative impact on your life. Everyday causes of excessive sweating include anxiety, eating spicy food, hot weather, exercise and certain medications. Conditions such as hyperhidrosis, where there are misfiring sympathetic nerves overstimulating the sweat glands, can cause excessive sweating too. Making sure you wear loose-fitting and breathable clothing, rather than tight-fitting clothes or leather, can definitely make a difference. Regularly showering and using an antiperspirant also help, as do relaxing techniques to reduce anxiety, such as yoga or meditation. If commercial deodorants are causing irritation, you could use antibacterial surgical scrub soaps which are available at pharmacies or mix baby powder and baking soda for gentle but effective protection. Sometimes seeking medical help can work and approved treatments like Botox injections, low-intensity electric currents and even surgery to remove sweat glands can be very beneficial when all else has failed.

Five ways to improve your hygiene

2

WASH OFF EXCESSIVE SWEAT IN THE SUMMER OR AFTER EXERCISE

Excessive sweat that you don't wash off can put you at high risk of sunburn, because when we sweat there is reduced ultraviolet light protection.

1

SHOWER DAILY

Poor hygiene can put you at risk of acne, eczema and psoriasis, and lead to dermatitis and developing patches of plaque on the skin. If you avoid daily showers because you are prone to skin irritation, try showering with cooler water. Just make sure you shower at least once a day and so reduce the chance of developing skin disease.

3

WASH YOUR HANDS REGULARLY

This has been drilled into us since the start of the coronavirus pandemic as a way to avoid infection and keep clean. We should be doing this after using the toilet with soap and water and when out and about with alcohol hand gel.

4

TRIM YOUR NAILS REGULARLY

This can help to avoid nail bed infections, in-growing nails and hang nails (a piece of hard, torn skin around the edge of the nail), and can prevent athletes' foot and other fungal infections.

5

MAKE SURE TO WIPE PROPERLY
(front to back)

After using the toilet and change to clean underwear regularly to avoid urinary and skin infections.

SMELLY FEET

I'm sure you've gathered by now that a lot of the embarrassing things that can happen to the human body have something to do with smell – and feet are no different! Sometimes smelly feet can be caused by hyperhidrosis, which is excessive sweating, or it could be from socks and shoes made of certain materials that cause your feet to sweat, so try changing your footwear. Using underarm antiperspirant on your feet or using a hairdryer on a cool setting to dry your toes after showering can also help. If these things don't make a difference, you may have a fungal or bacterial problem which may be causing the smell, in which case you should seek medical advice.

RECTAL ITCH

As well as embarrassing this can be very irritating and annoying, and there is nothing that can really ruin your day like an itchy booty. It can be caused by poor wiping or even a prolapsed rectum, and sometimes threadworms (pinworms), warts or haemorrhoids. It's important to make sure you're wiping well after a bowel movement and use unscented baby wipes rather than toilet paper if necessary. Using nappy rash ointment or antifungal powders before bedtime can also ease the itch.

If you have extreme itching around the anus or vagina, especially at night, you might have a case of threadworm. You can check this at home by sticking some sticky tape over your anus at night – the worms exiting your bottom will stick to the tape and thus you can identify why you might have the itch. You can then let your GP know and get the correct treatment.

FLATULENCE

Passing gas is a very natural thing for all of us, and can happen up to 20 times a day. Sometimes you can feel a bit gassier due to the stuff you eat, such as beans and lentils, or if you are drinking or eating high-sugar drinks or food. Sometimes even caffeinated drinks like coffee can cause excessive gas, as well as certain medications and antibiotics. If you can, try eating more slowly. If you're having problems with digestion, you can try over-the-counter products containing enzymes, like lactase supplement, before a meal. A lactase enzyme supplement helps the body digest the lactose in dairy products preventing pain, cramping, bloating, gas and diarrhoea. Try to avoid excessive consumption of problem foods, such as those that contain sulphur (meat, eggs and cauliflower for example) and sugary products – this is going to really help with the smell too!

CONSTIPATION

Constipation is very uncomfortable and many of us have suffered from it. It can be embarrassing and leave us a little bit red-faced when we can't get it out and get on with our day. Constipation can be caused by not drinking enough water, eating a low-fibre diet, inactivity, stress or certain medications for pain, among other things. Sometimes, as we get older, our pelvic floor muscles can weaken and this can make passing stools even more difficult, which means the large intestines have to work harder. Simple stuff like taking milk of magnesia or gentle over-the-counter laxatives can help. Exercising for 30 minutes a day and eating a good amount of fibre, or having a stimulant like coffee, can also help. There are a few medical causes for constipation, so if over-the-counter simple methods don't work, make sure to seek medical advice.

HOW TO PREVENT CONSTIPATION

- **increase your fibre intake**
- **get regular exercise and move around during the day**
- **make sure you're adequately hydrated and drinking enough water during the day**
- **try to open your bowels when you feel like it rather than holding it in**
- **have smaller and more regular meals**
- **increase the strength of your pelvic floor muscles by doing simple Kegel exercises (see page 67)**

Medical myth

WE ONLY USE 10 PER CENT OF OUR BRAINS

I'm not exactly sure where this one came from, however medical neurological studies have shown that we can identify the areas of the brain used for different functions. This is how we know that the different parts of the brain are responsible for doing different things. The brain is a very complicated structure and we definitely do not use only 10 per cent of it.

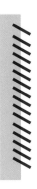

GENITAL INJURIES

A genital injury is an injury to the sex organs, mainly those outside the body. It refers to the area in between the legs called the perineum as well. Indeed, genital injuries can be very painful and cause a lot of bleeding. Sometimes injuries can affect the reproductive organs, the bladder and the urethra, and the damage caused can be temporary or permanent.

Children can get a genital injury by placing items into the vagina, having a toilet seat fall down on the genital area, getting it caught in a trouser zip or having a straddle injury (when the area between the legs is injured by perhaps falling onto a bike seat or the top of a fence) can lead to an A&E visit. And in adults genital injuries can result from sexual play or sexual pleasure, especially when using sexual paraphernalia.

If there's any severe bleeding, try to keep direct pressure on the wound and keep calm. Place a clean, sterile dressing on any open wounds. If the vagina is bleeding, place a clean cloth in the area. Apply cold compresses to reduce any swelling. Do not try to remove any objects yourself and seek medical help straightaway.

SEXUALLY TRANSMITTED INFECTIONS (STIS)

Having sex without protection can be risky business. You're leaving yourself open to STIs such as HIV and chlamydia and you're also risking potential unwanted pregnancy. Because of how common STIs are, it's very unsafe to have unprotected sex (sex without contraception or a condom) with multiple partners. You only have to have sex with someone once to catch one or more STI. Also, you can't tell whether somebody has an STI just by looking at them and so the best way to avoid infection is to use a condom every time you have sex.

Multiple STIs can lead to serious abdominal infections and sometimes can even cause infertility. Some types of oral sex are linked to the spread of human papillomavirus (HPV) infection, which can lead to cancer in the mouth and throat.

There are two types of emergency contraception: the intrauterine device (IUD, see page 76) or the emergency contraceptive pill, sometimes called the 'morning after' pill. There is advice on the NHS website about when to take emergency contraception after having unprotected sex.

How do I know if I have a STI and what should I do if I have one?

If you're worried about possibly having an STI it's important to go for a check-up at the sexual health clinic or see your GP as soon as you can. Symptoms can include:

- unusual discharge from the vagina, penis or anus
- pain when peeing
- a rash
- unusual vaginal bleeding
- an itchy anus hole or genitals
- warts and blisters around your genitals

The clinician will often take a full sexual history and may examine you. They will then run some more investigations or go ahead and treat you. If you are found to be positive for an STI, it's important to tell your ex- or current sexual partner(s) so they can get tested and treated as well.

WHAT'S THE BEST CONTRACEPTIVE TO USE?

This is an interesting question because there's such a wide range of different contraceptive methods available in the UK. Your best choice is likely to depend on your health and your circumstances. The main thing is to make sure you make an informed decision. Speak to your GP or sexual health clinic professional or look online at nhs.uk.

Contraceptives that are said to be 99 per cent effective include the contraceptive implant, the intrauterine system (IUS), the IUD or female sterilisation. For men, this includes male sterilisation or vasectomy. The IUS and IUD are both T-shaped devices that are inserted into the uterus by a medical professional. The IUS releases progestogen and the IUD is made from copper, which can help prevent you getting pregnant. The IUD is sometimes referred to as the 'coil'.

When used correctly, the contraceptive injection, the combined pill, the contraceptive patch, the vaginal ring or the progestogen-only pill can give up to 95 per cent protection. Contraceptives that can also protect you against STIs and disease include male and female condoms. Some people prefer to use natural family planning if they do not like barrier or hormonal protection. However, this does not protect you from contracting sexually transmitted diseases (STDs) or STIs and there are significantly more risks of unexpected pregnancy if not carried out correctly.

WHEN TO GO TO A&E

Wondering whether or not to go to the emergency department? If you have any of these symptoms, please go, go, go!

- **persistent chest pains**
- **difficulty breathing**
- **severe allergic reaction**
- **multiple traumatic injuries**
- **severe, uncontrollable bleeding**
- **head injury and loss of consciousness**
- **non-responsive baby**
- **severe burns or wounds**
- **acute confused state**
- **signs of a stroke: acute slurred speech, facial numbness, visual difficulties (see page 50)**

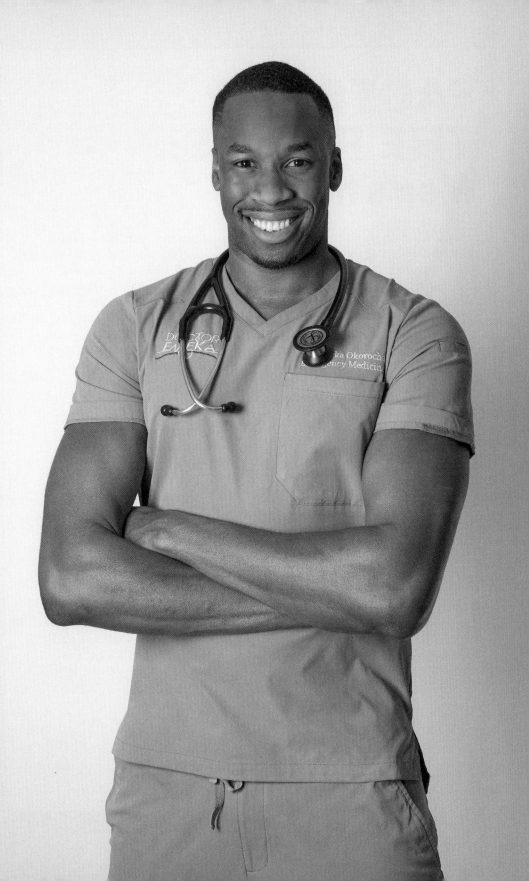

FACTS FOR THE FELLAS:
Men's health

So lads, when it comes to our health, history has shown that we're not exactly the best at taking care of it – whether this is feeling too embarrassed to go to the doctor when you have an issue, or thinking that you can heal your own wounds, or being too ashamed to open up about a slightly awkward condition or mental health concern. Studies have shown that men also don't go to the doctor because we don't like taking time off work and we go to the doctor a lot less than women. However, when men and women retire, they actually go to the doctor about the same amount of time. Shockingly, in the UK 1 man in every 5 dies before the age of 65 and 22 per cent of men in Scotland die before they even retire. So, while you may be working hard and hate the thought of taking time off, it's really important that you prioritise your physical and mental health – and take it seriously.

Men are 67 per cent more likely to die from the common cancers that affect both men and women (with the exception of breast cancer). Prostate cancer is the most common form of cancer amongst men (see pages 54–5), so if you have any urinary dysfunction, such as bleeding when you pee, or problems with ejaculation and erections, and even pain in the back passage, it's important to get checked by a doctor. There is a common misconception that breast cancer only affects women, but we are seeing numbers rising amongst men every year. So when we think of testicular cancer and checking your grapes downstairs, you should also be checking those percolating pectorals.

Diabetes (see page 50) is another common health problem that affects men, but that doesn't get much attention as a male problem because of the vast amount of people that it affects. However, men are twice as likely to die from diabetic complications than women. One of the huge risk factors for this is that men and boys are more likely to be overweight or obese than women or girls at the same age. This stresses just how important it is to establish good eating habits and have a balanced diet from an early age (see pages 94–117 for more on this).

I know men can be a little bit shy and reluctant to see the doctor. You may not admit it, but many of you have some common questions as I get asked them time and time again, both in A&E and through social media, so I've included them opposite:

WHAT MAKES MY PENIS SMELLY?

There are a number of common causes for a stinky, painful penis, such as:

STIS: these include gonorrhoea, which can cause unusual white, yellow or green discharge from the penis, or chlamydia, which can cause white, cloudy discharge from the penis and pain in the testicles when peeing, so make sure you protect yourself when you're having fun with your partner (see page 74).

URETHRITIS: this is inflammation of the urethra, which is a tube that runs from the bladder to the tip of the penis, and is often caused by a UTI. The symptoms are similar to a UTI – such as white or cloudy discharge from the tip of the penis, a burning sensation when you pee or a frequent need to pee – where an infection can develop in the whole of the urinary tract such as the bladder, urethra or even the kidneys.

SMEGMA: this is the cheesy-looking substance that builds up when you don't wash your penis properly. It's a natural lubricant that's found on the head of the penis under the foreskin and can be a breeding area for bacteria, so make sure you wash well.

BALANITIS: this can be caused by an infection or skin conditions such as psoriasis, and it's where the head of the penis becomes red and swollen. It could also be related to a build-up of smegma.

PROSTATITIS: this is a condition which results in inflammation of your prostate gland and can cause pain in the penis as well as the testicles, the tummy and the lower back, so make sure you seek medical advice if you think this is what you may have.

WHAT SHOULD I DO ABOUT LUMPS ON MY TESTICLES OR PENIS?

We regularly advise males to have a nice feel of their genitals in a warm, clean environment such as the shower at least once a month, and you might actually find some sort of lump, rash or skin change. Often these are not caused by anything serious, but you should always see your GP if you notice any changes or have any concerns.

When it comes to testicles, most are the same size but it's common for one to be bigger than the other or hang a little bit lower so you shouldn't be too concerned. The testicles should generally feel smooth without any lumps or bumps. However, you can feel a soft tube at the back of the testicle which is the epididymis (the tube that stores and carries sperm). Things to look out for when you examine yourself are a hard lump on the front or side of the testicle, a swelling or enlargement of the testicle or pain and discomfort in the scrotum. If you find any of these, it's important to make sure you get it checked out by a doctor as soon as possible.

CAUSES OF LUMPS AND BUMPS IN THE TESTES INCLUDE:

VARICOCELE: caused by large veins, which could look like a bag of worms and is often painless and fairly common. This might make one of your testicles feel heavier.

HYDROCELE: a visible swelling caused by fluid around the testicle making one appear much larger. Most of the time this is painless, but can leave you with a little discomfort if large enough.

EPIDIDYMAL CYST: a lump caused by fluid in the epididymis.

TESTICULAR TORSION: an acute, sudden, painful swelling that happens when a testicle becomes twisted. It often occurs with younger men or boys, but can affect you at a later age. This is a medical emergency – go to A&E as soon as possible.

EPIDIDYMITIS: an infection causing inflammation of the epididymis which can cause pain, swelling and tenderness in the scrotum. Sometimes if left untreated this can cause nausea, fever and vomiting.

INGUINAL HERNIA: a scrotal swelling or lump which is caused by weakness in the abdominal wall allowing abdominal contents like the intestines to cause a bulge.

TESTICULAR CANCER: an uncommon cause of lumps and relatively quite rare, accounting for just 1 per cent of cancers that occur in men. Around 2,300 men are diagnosed with testicular cancer each year in the UK. It tends to affect younger men, commonly aged 15–49. However, it's one of the most treatable types of cancer and, in England and Wales, 99 per cent of people survive for a year or more after being diagnosed and 98 per cent survive for five years and more after diagnosis.

LUMPS ON THE PENIS CAN BE CAUSED BY A VARIETY OF THINGS, INCLUDING:

PEARLY PENILE PAPULES: flesh-coloured lumps found on the end of the penis. Some people think that these can be caused by an STI or bad hygiene, but they can be idiopathic, meaning arising spontaneously with no specific medical cause.

FORDYCE SPOTS: yellowish white spots on the head or shaft of the penis. They can also occur inside the cheeks or on the lips as well and are generally harmless and do not require treatment.

PENILE CANCER: can cause a sore or lump on the penis or the head of the penis.

LYMPHOCELE: a hard swelling that suddenly appears on the shaft of the penis after sex or masturbation. This occurs when the lymph channels in the penis are temporarily blocked. Any swelling usually soon subsides and doesn't cause permanent problems.

LICHEN PLANUS: an itchy purple, non-infective rash.

GENITAL WARTS: small growths or bumps that appear on the shaft, or sometimes the head, of the penis or on the foreskin. These are actually caused by HPV – an STI.

OTHER STDS: sores or blisters on the head of the penis can be caused by the herpes simplex virus, or a painless sore or ulcer on the penis can be caused by syphilis.

MOLLUSCUM CONTAGIOSUM: a viral skin infection that can affect the penis and the groin area and is actually considered an STI as well.

I know it can be scary to possibly find a lump or bump down there, but it's better to check them than not to. You're far more likely to survive a potential testicular cancer when it's been caught early and hasn't spread to other parts of the body.

HOW CAN I INCREASE MY CHANCES OF HAVING A BABY?

When it comes to conception, aka producing babies, there are a couple of common factors at play. The first is how often you're having sex. It might seem a bit basic, but if you want a good chance of conception, you have to increase the amount of times you're having sex to at least two or three times a week. The second comes down to sperm and basically how viable it is. Your testicles are outside the body because they need to be cooler than the rest of your body for a good sperm temperature. So, if you find yourself getting hot and bothered down there, make sure you wear loose underwear, change it regularly and give your balls some air. This can help affect sperm temperature and cool things down.

Other lifestyle factors, such as smoking, can reduce fertility, so it's a good idea to stop. Drinking alcohol excessively can also reduce the quality of sperm so make sure you're not bingeing every week or exceeding the recommended 14 units a week, which should be spread over three days or more (see pages 32–7 for more on this). Recreational drugs, such as cannabis and cocaine, and anabolic steroids also affect your sperm quality. And actually some medication that we give in hospital – such as long-term antibiotics, chemotherapy and other drugs – can affect your sperm, so if you have any queries or concerns about what you're taking, speak to your doctor. It's also useful to know that having a healthy, balanced diet, maintaining a good weight and exercising regularly increase the chance of having a baby, so the health hacks I've included throughout this book will help too. Severe stress may also limit the production of sperm so try to take steps to relax and manage your stress (see page 188). Try all these tips and you should be on your way to having your own bouncing bundle of joy.

DOES SIZE REALLY MATTER, OR IS IT ALL IN OUR HEAD?

Men everywhere at some point worry about whether their penis is smaller than it should be or if it is satisfactory. Possibly due to media and pornography, men have always placed great importance on the size of their penis, and this has been associated with their masculinity. Sometimes when you're feeling inadequate, it can have a big impact on your confidence and your mental health and lead to relationship issues.

The internet and companies around the world have exploited all these issues by offering big boosting pills and extender products which promise to make your penis a mega mass machine by increasing its length and girth.

The average penis size is somewhere around 9cm long when not erect, and the erect size can be about 13–18cm. It's also key to note that your penis probably looks larger to other people, so try looking in the mirror rather than looking down. It's all about angles! It's also important to note that to a lot of partners size doesn't matter – very few have a massive interest in the size of their partner's penis and instead are focused on the connection they have with the person they're with. There is counselling available for men with penis anxiety which could be beneficial, but I suggest you concentrate more on building connection with your partner rather than the size of your tackle...

MEN'S MENTAL HEALTH

Men are more likely to die by suicide than women in the UK and men aged 40–49 actually have the highest suicide rate. Men in general report less self-satisfaction and are less likely to access psychological therapy and get help due to stigma and a number of socio-economic factors. Men are also far more likely to turn to coping strategies such as drug abuse and alcoholism to cope with deteriorating mental health, which ultimately will just make things worse. This is why I feel it's so important to include this section in this book – to stress just how important it is that poor male mental health needs to be identified and treated properly.

There is still a lot of stigma around men's mental health in society. Many men feel that they can't talk about their mental health problems because their peers will perceive them as weak. A lot of men feel under pressure to provide for themselves and their families, and any crack in their mental health or mental state can be seen as a 'failure'. It's sadly still common to hear phrases like 'man up' if a man talks about his feelings and men can often be dismissive of their colleagues, friends and family members when it comes to discussing and being open about mental health, stress, depression and anxiety. Men are often under the impression that they have to be completely self-reliant and take control of any situation, whether physical or mental.

However, just like if somebody comes to see me with a broken arm or leg in A&E and I tell them it is going to get better with medical intervention, mental health conditions like anxiety and depression can and will get better if you seek help.

On average, 12.5 per cent of males around the world will experience some sort of depression at some time in their life and almost 21 per cent will experience some sort of anxiety. Many symptoms can be physical, such as sweating, a racing heart, feeling sick or dizzy, and not being able to sleep. Emotional anxiety symptoms include catastrophic thinking, a feeling of impending doom, reduced concentration, avoidance and irritability. The problem is that men are less likely to seek help than women, and get worse and worse until the point where the presentation is quite severe, and this can often be linked to alcohol or substance abuse. Depression can then manifest itself with feeling very low and not being able to involve yourself in tasks you love, a change in eating pattern and loss of sex drive, and in extreme cases feeling suicidal.

It's really important that when these symptoms are identified you seek help. It's also vital that we recognise these signs and symptoms in the men around us and encourage them to talk to someone about what they're experiencing. There are many subtle things you can do to encourage the important males in your life to make daily lifestyle choices which can help them reduce their stress and anxiety, and prevent depression from progressing, such as keeping them active during the day, helping them make an action plan and engaging them in activities they enjoy or once enjoyed, usually with friends.

Similarly, there are lots of ways to reduce your own stress and anxiety and increase your mood and confidence:

- **looking after your body through physical activity**
- **eating a healthy diet**
- **getting a good night's sleep**

The avoidance of alcohol, drug and substance abuse is also imperative for good mental health. It may make you feel a little bit better in the short term; however, it will be very detrimental in the long term.

In society we need to reduce the stigma around talking to our mates or professionals about our mental health, which leads to us bottling things up. All of us should be taking our mental health very seriously.

THE MALE MENOPAUSE

The male menopause is a phenomenon that men can experience which can refer to depression, loss of sex drive, erectile dysfunction and physical and emotional symptoms in their late forties and early fifties. Common symptoms include:

- **mood swings and irritability**
- **loss of muscle mass**
- **general lack of enthusiasm and energy**
- **difficulty sleeping**
- **poor concentration**
- **fat redistribution, such as getting a large belly or 'man boobs'**

Ordinarily, testosterone levels fall gradually in a steady decline as people age, which doesn't necessarily manifest with problems. However, the above symptoms tend to be due to a sudden drop in testosterone in middle age. Lifestyle factors and psychological problems – generally brought on by work, relationship issues or money problems – can often result in symptoms and can lead to stress, depression and anxiety. This could also be referred to as a 'midlife crisis' when men have reached the halfway stage of life.

If you're experiencing these symptoms it's good to talk to your GP who may take a medical history, ask about your personal life and investigate whether your symptoms are affected by or caused by anything else. Your GP may also test your blood and measure your testosterone levels to check for any deficiency, and if there is any identified it can be treated with tablets, patches or injections.

Foods that can boost your testosterone!

- **oysters**
- **pomegranates**
- **soya milk**
- **beans**
- **ginger**
- **honey**
- **spinach**

BODY DYSMORPHIA

Most eating disorders are found in women, perhaps because women talk more about food and dieting due to societal expectations placed on women's bodies. In addition, weight loss in women who are dieting can be seen a lot earlier, whereas men may mask this with excessive exercise or going to the gym. Men are also likely to avoid seeking help because they may be stigmatised. However, men and boys can suffer from eating disorders, and those men who do often care more about what their friends or other people think, which can present as male body dysmorphia.

Triggers for eating problems with men may include:

- **being bullied for being overweight**
- **negative comments from an athletics or sports coach**
- **illness**
- **loss or bereavement at home**
- **social media stigma**
- **relationship breakdown**
- **not coping with pressures such as exams**
- **a career change or difficulties with pressures at work**

It's important to try to treat the cause of the issue and seek help where appropriate.

MY TOP FIVE TIPS FOR MEN TO KEEP MENTALLY HEALTHY

1. **Don't be afraid to be vulnerable: talk to someone close or a health professional if you are feeling unwell or stressed.**
2. **Try to find some form of daily exercise that works for you: this will not only help physically but mentally too.**
3. **Stay connected: make sure you surround yourself with family and friends who make you happy or join new groups and clubs.**
4. **Get a good night's sleep and eat a healthy, balanced diet.**
5. **Have a regular check-up with your GP: looking after your physical health is key to staying mentally healthy.**

THE LOWDOWN FOR THE LASSES:
Women's health

Now ladies, this section is all about your health and you and your body. We know that in general women are better at being mindful about taking care of their health than their male counterparts, but there are a number of different things that females can go through medically that men can never truly understand or experience for themselves. So, in this section, speaking as a doctor, I'm going to try to give you some info that you can use. After all, like Beyoncé once said, Who runs the world? Girls!

While women tend to be more conscious of their health, they spend more time suffering from chronic disease. Some of these reasons may be classed as physiological, some as behavioural and some as environmental as women are often more likely to be caregivers and under more stress and therefore require more support both physically and mentally.

There are certain diseases which affect both men and women, but that more commonly occur in women, such as asthma, arthritis, rheumatism, fibromyalgia and lupus. And we haven't even mentioned the fact that women have female reproductive systems containing ovaries, fallopian tubes, uteruses and vaginas, which means they can be at risk of conditions such as heavy menstrual bleeding, bacterial vaginosis, endometriosis, ovarian disease, vulval disease and gynaecological cancers.

However, as difficult as it may be being a lady, there are many things that are said to be in women's favour when it comes to health. Females tend to live longer than their male counterparts, and many believe this could be due to the fact that women have stronger immune systems and are better at fighting off infections. Studies suggest that the female hormone oestrogen plays a good part in curbing the expression of an enzyme that hinders the body's defence system against bacterial viruses, though researchers aren't exactly sure why. One theory is that this comes down to the role of giving birth and nursing offspring. Studies also show that women have better memory skills than men because they unconsciously spend more time studying new faces and also tend to remember things on lists better than men.

EATING DISORDERS

Eating disorders are more prevalent in women than men. Eating disorders can include anorexia or bulimia and are caused by a number of different things, but they often stand alongside a psychological condition. Like any kind of disease, eating disorders, if left untreated, will only get worse, which is why it's good to identify if you or someone you know is struggling. Behaviours such as making yourself vomit after meals, inducing diarrhoea with laxatives or binge eating during a specific situation when you're not even hungry could be a sign you have an eating disorder.

We've established how complex the female body is, so it's not surprising that a lot of women have many questions to ask about their bodies when going to the doctor. I've included the most common ones over the next few pages:

HOW CAN I INCREASE MY CHANCES OF GETTING PREGNANT?

Pregnancy happens when sperm enters the vagina and fertilises a viable female egg – simple in principle, but a very complicated web depending on so many different factors, and health does play a big part. Certain lifestyle changes, such as maintaining a healthy weight, stopping or reducing alcohol consumption and smoking – both you and your partner – and taking folic acid every day can increase your chances of conception. Cutting back on caffeine and getting regular exercise helps too.

Make sure you're having sex every 2–3 days without using contraception so the sperm actually enters the vagina and try to have regular sex around the time when you're ovulating. Ovulation is when an egg is released from one of your ovaries. To work out when you're ovulating, you can look at the length of your menstrual cycle. Ovulation often occurs around 10–16 days before your period starts. Sometimes you can notice a change in your cervical mucus as it may be wetter, clearer and more slippery around the time of ovulation. You can identify ovulation by your body temperature, as there is a small rise when ovulation takes place, and you can also get uncomfortable abdominal pain. Your hormone levels also increase around the time of ovulation and this can be detected using a simple at-home ovulation predictor kit. There are also some amazing apps available that track your cycle and can be really useful for family planning.

If you're under the age of 40 and have regular sex without using contraception, there is an 80 per cent chance that you'll be pregnant within a year. A healthy 30-year-old woman having regular unprotected sex 2–3 times a week has a 20 per cent chance of falling pregnant each month.

IF I'VE HAD AN ABORTION, WILL IT AFFECT MY FERTILITY?

Understandably, if you've had an abortion you might have some concerns about your fertility. However, there is no medical evidence that states that having an abortion reduces your chances of becoming pregnant or having normal pregnancies in the future. However, if during the abortion you develop a womb infection that is not then treated properly, that's when there could be a small risk of infertility for future pregnancy. Pelvic inflammatory disease (PID) is a condition caused by an infection which can possibly increase your risk of infertility or ectopic pregnancy. In England, Scotland and Wales we carry out abortions legally before 24 weeks of pregnancy, or sometimes after in very limited circumstances when the mother's life is at risk. There are many reasons you may want to carry out an abortion and you should remember that the decision is yours and yours alone, and you should speak to your GP, a specialist or the counselling service at the abortion clinic for help and advice. Be mindful that this is a personal decision that you shouldn't feel guilty about. It can also be useful to discuss this with your partner, family or friends; however, always remember that you have the final decision.

WHAT CAN I DO TO EASE PAINFUL PERIODS?

There are so many different causes of pain during periods and the painful sensation differs between people. Some medical causes include endometriosis, fibroids or even PID. And for some people it's just a very painful experience because the muscular wall of the womb tightens and contracts and can cause severe cramping. This can become normal for your menstrual cycle and most people will experience it at some point in their lives. The best way to treat period pain at home is with over-the-counter painkillers such as ibuprofen or aspirin. However, if you have asthma, or stomach, kidney or liver problems, you should speak to your GP about what painkillers you should take. You can also try paracetamol; however, for some women this might not be strong enough to fully reduce the pain. Sometimes your GP can even prescribe stronger painkillers such as codeine or naproxen. It's also useful to talk to your GP about contraceptives as these can ease period pain. Lifestyle measures that can alleviate period pain are stopping smoking and partaking in regular exercise. Sometimes using a heat pad or hot water bottle, or taking a warm bath can ease cramps, and having a light massage can help as well.

WHY DO I SOMETIMES BLEED BETWEEN PERIODS?

Bleeding between periods can be down to many different reasons. Often it's nothing to worry about, especially if it's light spotting; however, if you're concerned you should seek medical advice. Sometimes bleeding can occur in the first few months of starting new hormonal contraception. Other causes include injury to the vagina and having penetrative sex, recently having an abortion, STIs or STDs, or recent miscarriage. Sometimes bleeding can be due to vaginal dryness and in older ladies it can even be a sign of cancer. If you are concerned about bleeding between your periods you should see your GP or attend a sexual health clinic.

WHAT IS MENOPAUSE AND WHAT SYMPTOMS SHOULD I LOOK OUT FOR?

Menopause occurs in women when they have their last menstrual period. We define a woman as 'postmenopausal' when they haven't had a period for over a year. However, menopause can take several years to go through as periods become less and less frequent. This is a natural process that all women will go through as they age, and it occurs as the ovaries stop producing eggs and make less oestrogen. The average age of women going through menopause in the UK is 51.

Common symptoms of menopause include:

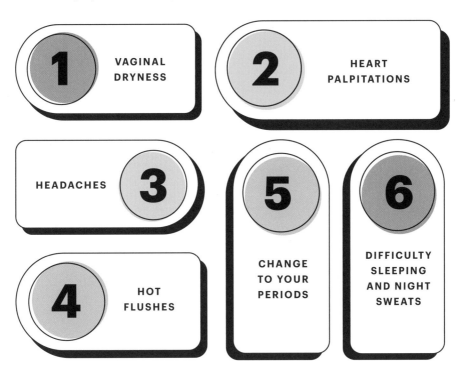

1 VAGINAL DRYNESS

2 HEART PALPITATIONS

HEADACHES 3

5 CHANGE TO YOUR PERIODS

6 DIFFICULTY SLEEPING AND NIGHT SWEATS

4 HOT FLUSHES

Many women are aware of the hormonal changes that can occur during menopause and what the physical changes and symptoms may be. However, many women aren't aware that the menopause can also affect their mental health. Menopause comes with new symptoms such as irritability, and the feeling of sadness, lack of motivation and an increase in anxiety and stress. This can cause emotional strain and affect your mental health which can increase your chances of developing depression. Other external factors occurring at the same time as the menopause can also contribute to poor mental health, such as concerns about the health of your parents or partner while they also age, or having problems with relationships, life expectations and occupation. Often we treat symptoms of menopause with hormone replacement therapy (HRT), replacing the oestrogen in the body. This can be in the form of creams, sprays, tablets, patches or vaginal rings. Although this may have benefits for the symptoms of menopause, it also may have risks so it's important to speak to your doctor if you would like more information.

IS IT NORMAL TO FEEL WORRIED OR ANXIOUS ALL THE TIME?

When it comes to mental health, social and economic factors play such a huge part, probably more so for women than for men. Women generally find it easier to express themselves and talk about their feelings; however, 1 in 5 women in the UK still report experiencing common mental health problems, such as depression anxiety, and there can be many different reasons for this. Women may have experienced sexual violence or sexual abuse, they may have post-traumatic stress disorder (PTSD) or they may be concerned about their personal safety and well-being, or that of their children and families, which can lead to struggles with mental health issues. Women go through life-changing experiences that men don't, such as pregnancy and giving birth – which can develop into perinatal depression, also known as the 'baby blues' – or menopause, which I cover in more detail above. Hormones play a huge part in how we feel and women have changes in their hormones every month. These factors can contribute to a deterioration in mental health.

'

If you're worried about your mental health, the best thing to do is to talk to somebody – whether this is a support network online, a family member or your GP. It's important that people know what you're going through and how they can help you to get through it, so please don't be afraid to reach out.

,

SWIT

HC

SWIT

CH

TIW a

CH UP YOUR DIET

SWITCH UP YOUR DIET

'

MOTIVATION

It's raining, it's gloomy, you haven't slept... but, guess what, none of that matters! It's those times when you have setbacks, when things aren't looking good and yet you still have that burning desire to get up and do what you do and chase your goals that make the greats great. Remember your 'why' and use that when times get rough. Tunnel vision all the way to the top!

'

I'm sure by now everyone knows that resolving many health issues revolves around improving your diet. But we've all seen people trying different fad diets and making New Year's resolutions and having difficulty sticking to them, and it can be hard to know what a healthy, balanced diet actually looks like. The key to a good diet is consistency and making small, doable changes that you can realistically achieve. Crash dieting for a holiday or an event isn't the way forward and will end up making you feel worse than when you started – it's a poisoned chalice destined for failure.

Now, I'm a doctor, not a dietician, but I am a huge advocate for healthy eating and have done some of my own research into how to make my meals more nutritious and improve my diet, so this chapter contains some of the quick diet hacks that I've used that can help you too, but first let's cover the basics of healthy eating.

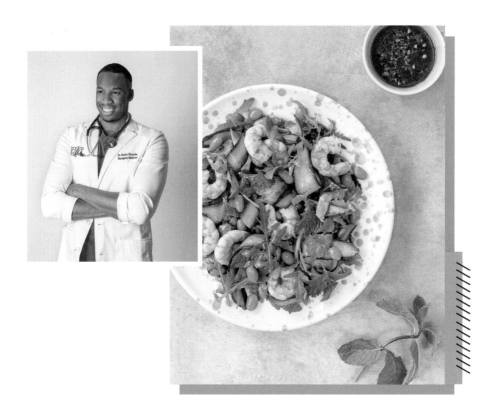

Nutrition basics

Food is integral to our health and longevity, but what do we mean by a balanced diet and how do you sort the facts from the fads? A healthy diet is one where you consume the quantities that you expend. It should be balanced with all the essential dietary nutrients, proteins, vitamins and minerals that the body needs, and it should give you energy and adequate nutrition.

When it comes to nutrition, a lot of us don't understand exactly how much we should be getting from our food. It's therefore important to note that nutritional values are often labelled clearly on food products and packages. For example, the traffic light system of colour-coding helps us to see at a glance whether the food is high (red), medium (amber) or low (green) in fat, saturated fat, sugars and salt, so it's always worth keeping your wits about you when you're grabbing those bargains at the supermarket.

The daily reference intakes (RIs; the maximum amount of nutrients you should eat on average in a day) for a fully grown adult are:

TOTAL FAT	less than 70g
SATURATES	less than 20g
CARBOHYDRATE	260g
TOTAL SUGARS	90g
PROTEIN	50g
SALT	less than 6g

KEEP A FOOD LOG

Try to track and keep a log of the food you eat. A lot of us munch so much we sometimes don't realise just how much we're eating! Keeping a log makes you consciously aware of what you're consuming so you can cut it down if you need to. You may find it useful to use an app to track what you're eating and how many calories you take in during the day if you're short on time.

Now, everyone is different and one size certainly does not fit all, so these values may vary depending on how active you are, how much you weigh and how fast your metabolism is, and they are not meant to be definitive targets. They just give a rough idea of how much you should be getting each day and what is deemed safe. We'll go through each of these in turn on the following pages and I'll share some of my one-minute hacks for a healthy, balanced diet.

HOW MANY CALORIES SHOULD I BE EATING PER DAY?

This is going to vary from person to person depending on how many calories you burn per day, your age, weight, size and body composition, and how active you are. But the daily threshold for the average size man and woman to maintain weight is about 2,000 calories for women and 2,500 calories for men. In medicine, we have a number of different equations that we can use to calculate and approximate recommended calories. It's also worth noting that these calories shouldn't be coming from one single source and your diet should be balanced, but more on that on next!

Not all fats are created equal

The body needs fat for a number of different processes. Fat helps the absorption of vitamins like A, D, E and K as they are fat-soluble and the body can only absorb them in the presence of fat. A lack of fat can cause deficiencies in these vitamins. Fat also supports cell growth, wound healing and hormone production, as well as providing us with energy.

SIGNS YOU MAY BE FAT-DEFICIENT

- difficulty adjusting vision at night
- swollen gums
- infertility
- muscle pain
- depression
- easy bruising
- dry hair
- dermatitis
- frequent sickness
- poor wound healing

One-minute diet hack

THROW OUT THE JUNK FOOD!

If, like me, you're easily tempted, don't put yourself in situations where you're going to snack on junk food.

There are several different types of fat:

TRANS FATS are unhealthy dietary fats that can raise cholesterol levels and the body just doesn't need them. These are found in processed and fried foods containing partially hydrogenated vegetable oil and increase your risk of heart disease and stroke.

SATURATED FATS tend to be solid at room temperature and are found in animal products like meat, eggs and dairy products, as well as chocolate, biscuits, pastries and cakes. Excessive consumption of these can raise your cholesterol and lead to heart disease.

MONOUNSATURATED FATS are fats that can reduce the LDL ('bad') cholesterol in the blood and this can reduce your chances of heart disease and stroke. These are liquid at room temperature and can be found in plant-based oils, some nuts and nut butters, and avocados.

POLYUNSATURATED FATS are known as 'essential fats' and include omega-3 fatty acids, which can help to reduce heart disease. Your body can't make these so it's important to include small amounts in your diet. You can find these in oysters, flaxseeds, chia seeds, soya beans, walnuts, eggs and oily fish. Omega-6 fatty acids are also essential and obtainable from our diet. They are found in rapeseed, corn and sunflower oil, and nuts. Most people get enough omega-6 in their diet and it plays a key role in providing us with energy and helps the immune system. However, too much can increase the risk of inflammation and inflammatory disease, so we should be eating more omega-3 than omega-6!

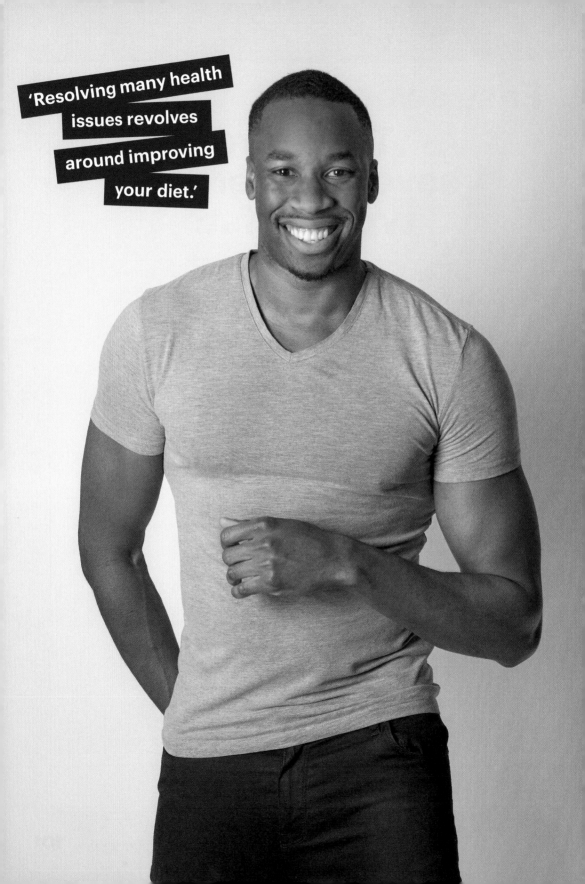

'Resolving many health issues revolves around improving your diet.'

Easy swaps

The decisions we make when it comes to eating will play a big part in how we are physically. This could be swapping highly calorific food for healthier options, or just changing how we cook our food – so grilling chicken rather than frying it.

TRY THIS...	INSTEAD OF THIS...
A PIECE OF FRUIT	A CHOCOLATE BAR
STILL/SPARKLING WATER	A CAN OF FIZZY DRINK
A FRESH SALAD	A BURGER
HOMEMADE SOUP	A PIZZA
A FRUIT SMOOTHIE	A MILKSHAKE
SOME VEGETABLE STICKS	A PLATE OF CHIPS
A PORTION OF NUTS/SEEDS	A PACKET OF CRISPS

One-minute diet hack

BE ADVENTUROUS

Try a new fruit or vegetable each week and you might come across something different that you really like.

Getting your five-a-day

The five-a-day rule comes from a campaign from the WHO, which recommends at a minimum that we should be consuming a variety of about 400g of fruit and vegetables per day to reduce the risk of serious health problems, such as cancer, stroke and heart disease.

A portion of fruit and vegetables is about 80g and you should be having roughly five varied portions per day. This could be a small portion of fruit at breakfast, like two small-sized fresh fruits such as satsumas or plums, an apple, banana or just a big old slice of melon or pineapple along with some veggie sticks at lunchtime and a couple of broccoli florets and some carrots or green beans with your main meal for dinner.

It might be easier to remember five reasons to have your five-a-day – these will hopefully stay in your mind and act as a prompt!

1. **They are delicious and there's so much variety to choose from – eating your five-a-day is a no-brainer!**
2. **They can help reduce your risk of heart disease and cancer.**
3. **They contribute to a healthy, balanced diet.**
4. **They are an excellent source of dietary fibre which may help maintain a healthy gut, ease digestive problems and reduce the risk of bowel cancer.**
5. **Fruit and vegetables are great sources of vitamin C, potassium and a number of different vitamins and minerals and are very nutritious!**

Medical myth

CARROTS GIVE YOU BETTER VISION

The basis of this rumour is that carrots contain carotene which the body then uses to make vitamin A, which helps maintain good vision. But the big catch here is that vitamin A is a fat-soluble vitamin that needs to be consumed with fat to be absorbed for the true benefits. So I'm afraid that eating a bunch of carrots on its own isn't going to give you night vision!

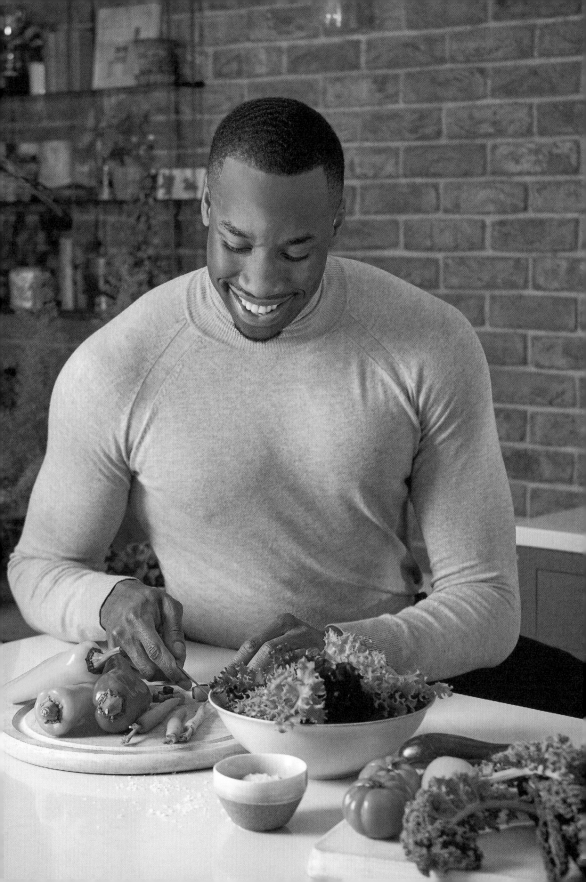

Carbs: good or bad?

The trend for low-carb diets and the whole business of labelling carbs as 'bad' has left a lot of people confused about carbohydrates and how important they are for our health. Carbs are an essential requirement in our diet. They are a great source of energy – containing fibre, calcium, iron and B vitamins. Gram for gram they contain fewer than half the calories of fat! Eating a healthy amount of carbs has also been known to provide good bowel health and reduce the risk of constipation, cardiovascular disease, type 2 diabetes and bowel cancer. However, the term 'carbohydrates' is a broad category and not all carbs are created equal. It all comes down to the type, the quantity and quality of the carbs we are eating.

The three main types of carbohydrate in food are sugars, starch and fibre. Our body breaks down carbs into glucose before absorbing them into the blood and, in this way, carbs make up the body's main source of energy. So ideally we should be eating starchy foods every day as part of a healthy, balanced diet. Foods such as potatoes, bread, rice, pasta and cereals should make up over a third of the food that we eat. Where possible, we should substitute white carbs for wholegrain varieties to up our fibre intake too. On average, most adults get about 19g of fibre a day, but the recommended fibre intake is about 30g a day. This is important to maintain good gut motility, and a diet high in fibre is also linked to reducing heart disease, stroke and bowel cancer, and can also prevent constipation.

Despite the promises of many fad diets, it would be very difficult to eliminate carbs from our diet because they are the body's main source of energy. In their absence, the body will break down protein and fat for energy and this is the basis of the 'keto' diet, which puts the body into a state of ketosis – the body will burn fat for energy. How healthy this diet can be is still under question and you may not be getting all the nutrients you need. Also, diets very high in proteins and fats can lead to issues with your kidneys and heart. In essence, for a healthy diet we should be eating carbohydrates that are high in fibre – and wholegrain where possible – in all our meals.

LOW-CARB DIETS AND DIABETES

If you're looking to start a low-carb diet and you have type 2 diabetes, you should speak to your GP because, although it's often safe when done well, drastically reducing or completely cutting out carbohydrates isn't suitable for everyone with type 2 diabetes as it can cause low blood sugar (hypoglycaemia).

Are fad diets just hype?

People are lured into fad diets in the same way as they are get-rich-quick schemes. And just like these schemes, fad diets often don't work. A number of different diets portray unrealistic and even dangerous results which can lead to nutritional disorders, yo-yo dieting and relapse. Like those scales you may dread standing on every morning at home, your diet should be perfectly balanced. Making small, realistic, achievable, gradual changes in your diet and using some of the smart swaps in this book are far more likely to lead to a sustainable, healthier diet and positive physical results.

Some sugary sense

You don't need excess sugar because you're sweet enough! Now, I'm a bit of a foodie and a sucker for anything sweet, seasoned or just great-tasting in general. But as a medical doctor I'm aware of just how important it is to regulate our sugar intake. The excess sugars that can lead to weight gain and poor dental hygiene are referred to as 'free sugars' and these are the ones we want to avoid. These excess, refined sugars are often added into our foods and drinks and are a major component in some of our favourite foods, such as biscuits, cake, chocolate and ready meals, and are found in things like fizzy drinks, syrups, honey and fruit juices. The sugars found naturally in stuff like milk, fruit and vegetables don't count as free sugars.

The government recommends that adults shouldn't be having more than 30g of free sugars per day, which is roughly about 7 sugar cubes. And children aged 7–10 shouldn't be having more than 24g of free sugars a day, which is about 6 sugar cubes. Younger children aged 4–6 shouldn't be having more than 19g of free sugars a day, which is about 5 sugar cubes.

I know what you're thinking, this sounds like a lot and there's no way you have this much. However, even a can of regular cola can have up to 9 cubes of sugar, which is more than the recommended daily limit for adults. And how many of us have had more than one can in a day?!

It's so important to look at the labels on our foods because some of the big offenders are our favourites:

- chocolate spread
- plain/milk/white chocolate
- sweets
- cola and other fizzy drinks
- squash
- sweetened fruit juice
- biscuits, buns and cakes
- doughnuts
- alcoholic drinks
- fruit yoghurt
- ice cream
- sweetened tea and coffee

Even savoury foods, such as salad cream and tomato ketchup, contain added sugars. If you can, try to cut down or even cut out refined sugar for one week and see if you can feel the benefits.

Six sugar busting tips

1
Swap sugary or fizzy drinks with water or unsweetened fruit juices and smoothies, though try not to have more than 150ml of juice a day.

2
If you prefer a fizzy drink, try mixing no added sugar squash with some sparkling water.

3
Try replacing your normal jam and spreads with reduced sugar versions.

4
Have fruit for dessert as it contains natural, rather than refined sugars and choose tinned fruit in juice rather than syrup. Hey, I'm just trying to keep you trim and healthy!

5
Check the nutrition labels when you're out food shopping and go for those foods with no added sugar.

6
Try unsweetened wholegrain breakfast cereals that are not frosted or coated with chocolate or honey.

Protein

Proteins are the building blocks of life. This is because they break down into amino acids that help our body grow and repair, so they're essential for building muscle mass and maintaining our metabolism.

Most of us in the UK actually eat twice as much protein as we need per day. The Department of Health advises adults not to consume more than twice the recommended daily amount of protein, which is 55.5g for men and 45g for women. Consuming too much protein can lead to an increased risk of osteoporosis, which is a disease that causes your bones to be brittle and places you at higher risk for a fracture, or it can worsen kidney problems. It's also important to know where our protein is coming from and that it's combined with carbohydrates, natural sugars and good fats throughout the day. Natural high-protein foods include meat (beef, lamb, pork and chicken), fish, eggs, dairy, beans, tofu and nuts.

One-minute diet hack

CHOOSE YOUR PROTEINS WISELY

Stats and studies have shown that eating a diet with increased red meat is associated significantly with cancer mortality and cardiovascular disease. Try eating lean, white meat, such as chicken, or have oily fish, nuts or pulses instead.

GETTING 'HENCH'

Now, I know that for many, when we think protein we think of building mega muscles! Protein supplements – in the form of powder, shakes, bars and capsules – are a standard part of the diet for many gym goers to help build and maintain body tissue and muscle. Many people also take amino acids which are known as the building blocks for muscle growth. Users tend to take supplementation before, during and even after training to enhance performance and improve recovery.

However, it should be noted that although protein shakes are convenient, they shouldn't be used as a meal replacement and you can get some of the same benefits from a protein-rich diet or even using snacks to add to your normal meals. Any extra protein should be supplementing a balanced diet not replacing it.

BEWARE: STEROIDS ARE SILLY

Doctors use steroids for various things in medicine and there are many different kinds. However, the illegal market anabolic steroids that people purchase in order to get hench may actually be harming their health. They are based on the male hormone testosterone and can therefore improve endurance and stimulate muscle growth.

HOWEVER, THEY CAN ALSO CAUSE:

- **an increase in blood pressure**
- **direct heart, kidney and liver damage**
- **acne**
- **a change in mood and increasing aggression**
- **sexual promiscuity**
- **reduced sperm count**
- **infertility**
- **breast development**
- **increased risk of prostate cancer**

Looking ripped is a goal for so many of us. However, at the end of the day, this can be achieved naturally and safely through techniques such as regular exercise and following a balanced diet. So, there's no need to ever put your health at risk to achieve a specific look.

One-minute diet hack

TRICK YOUR BRAIN

Use a smaller plate and trick your brain into thinking you're eating more.

Salt

Many of us want a lot more flavour in our food and so we can be guilty of adding too much salt to our meals. However, the increase in sodium can actually lead to a number of different conditions, such as high blood pressure, which then in turn can increase your risk of ischaemic heart disease, myocardial infarction (heart attack), stroke and cancer. We shouldn't be eating more than 6g of salt a day, which is 1 teaspoon. Make sure you check the salt content on cooked foods and meals you buy and watch how much salt you use in your own cooking. Try maybe adding a spice, pepper, herbs or alternative seasoning to get some extra flavour rather than salt.

Drink up

When people think about a healthy diet they often forget about water. We should be drinking at least 2.5 litres of water a day for women and 3.5 litres for men, depending on losses, temperature and activity. Try to have a glass of water with every meal and substitute soft drinks, juice or alcohol with water. And always, always make sure you drink plenty of water during exercise.

DON'T DRINK YOUR CALORIES

Just because you're not chewing it, it doesn't mean it isn't having an impact!

One-minute diet hack

EAT MINDFULLY

Try not to eat while you're watching TV or on the computer as you're far more likely to overeat. Being mindful of exactly what you're eating means that you won't eat for the sake of it, rather just when you're hungry, and you're more likely to be sure you're getting a balanced diet and hitting your targets on a range of food groups.

How do I know if I'm drinking enough water?

Many people are dehydrated and don't realise it. Some of the common signs of dehydration are:

- increased thirst
- very concentrated pee
- excessive dizziness
- fatigue
- dry mouth, eyes or lips

You can also get frequent headaches and this may be due to clinical dehydration. It's important that you keep hydrated, especially in the summer months when dehydration can lead to heat exhaustion and, even worse, heat stroke.

Is it worth taking vitamin pills?

Vitamin and mineral supplementation isn't always required, especially if you're getting your supplements from natural sources.

VITAMIN C

Helps with maintaining good skin and wound healing. You can find this in citrus fruits, potatoes and peppers.

VITAMIN A

Good for the skin and the body's immune system and also helps us to see in dim light. It can be found in cheese, oily fish, milk and yoghurt, and you can get it in good sources of beta-carotene such as leafy vegetables, carrots and yellow fruits like mango and apricots.

B VITAMINS

Useful for maintaining a healthy nervous system and providing energy. There are many types of B vitamin and they can be found in peas, nuts, milk, eggs, bread and liver. Folate is a B vitamin and the manmade form is folic acid. This helps produce red blood cells and reduces birth defects in pregnancy, and can be found in green leafy vegetables and broccoli. We recommend that pregnant women and women trying to conceive take 400 micrograms of folic acid every day in supplement form until 12 weeks pregnant.

CALCIUM

Essential for good bone strength and to help muscles move. Your body needs adequate calcium for your heart, nerves and muscles to function properly. It is found in milk, cheese and other dairy foods, alternative fortified milks and green leafy vegetables.

IRON

Needed for growth and development and to make haemoglobin, which is the component of the red blood cells that carries oxygen around the body, and myoglobin, which provides oxygen to your muscles. Iron is found in liver, red meat, beans and nuts.

VITAMIN D

Helps keep bones, teeth and muscles strong by regulating calcium and phosphate in the body. It is obtained naturally from direct sunlight and can also be found in oily fish, egg yolks and red meat. However, if you are found to be deficient, you may need added supplementation.

VITAMIN K

Essential for blood-clotting and helping wounds heal. Because of these properties, we use it and prescribe it in the emergency department. It is found in green leafy vegetables.

We can find all these vitamins and minerals naturally, which is recommended; however, we can also obtain them in supplement form such as a multivitamin. Please be aware, though, as we saw with the protein shakes used by gym goers, multivitamins are not a substitute for healthy, balanced meals.

Top tips for a balanced diet

2

VARIETY

Eat a variety of protein, such as beans, pulses, fish, eggs, meat and tofu.

1

CHECK YOUR FAT, SALT AND SUGAR

Try to reduce your fat, salt and sugar intake because fat and sugars contain a lot of calories but don't actually provide very many nutrients. Excessive consumption of fatty and sugary foods can cause unnecessary weight gain and increase the number of chronic health conditions you may have. Fast food and sugary drinks, as much as we crave them, can actually shorten our lifespan!

3

GET IN YOUR OILY FATS

Aim to eat at least two portions of fish a week, one of which should be oily fish, such as salmon or mackerel.

4

HIT YOUR FIVE-A-DAY

Eat at least five portions of a variety of fruit and vegetables per day.

5

TRY LOW FAT

Have some lower fat or lower sugar dairy options, such as soya drinks or yoghurts.

6

EAT YOUR CARBS

Base meals on potatoes, bread, rice, pasta or starchy carbohydrates and choose wholegrain or high-fibre versions where possible.

Food poisoning

Food poisoning is a usually short-lived illness that you get after you've ingested food or drink contaminated by germs and toxins. In the medical field we refer to this as 'gastroenteritis', which is basically an infection of the gut. Symptoms include vomiting, diarrhoea and tummy ache. You're likely to become dehydrated if you've been vomiting a lot and have diarrhoea and are not eating or drinking much, and this can produce symptoms such as tiredness, headaches, passing less urine and weakness. Make sure you hydrate yourself with simple fluids such as water.

If you're not able to keep anything down and you feel you're getting severely dehydrated, you have blood in your stools, are pregnant, have travelled abroad recently, are having severe pain and fevers which don't settle with simple over-the-counter medicine or have any other unfamiliar symptoms you're concerned about, you should seek medical advice. Symptoms usually settle within a few days as your immune system often clears the infection. This is another good reason why you need a healthy immune system!

FIVE WAYS TO PREVENT FOOD POISONING

1. Wash your hands and work surfaces before, during and after handling or preparing food.
2. Separate raw meat from other foods.
3. Ensure food is cooked all the way through to ensure any harmful bacteria are killed.
4. Make sure your fridge is kept at below 5°C.
5. Cool any leftovers quickly.

THAT
GUT
FEELING

MOTIVATION

I'm a big believer in continuous improvement, and I think a huge part of that is working on areas where you can be better.

We get gut instincts and gut feelings and we even sometimes get the 'bubble guts' when we are nervous. However, a lot of people don't realise just how important the gut is for keeping healthy and ensuring optimum physical and mental well-being.

The gut is made up of the microbiome, which is essential for human development, immunity and nutrition. It is a collection of microorganisms, such as different bacteria, viruses and fungi, which play a pivotal role in digesting the food we eat and absorbing the nutrients. The gut is made up of literally trillions of cells. They can be as unique as your fingerprint and can differ between identical twins. They're affected by the different cultures and the different types of food we eat.

Having a good overall healthy gut is vital; some professionals actually consider it almost as important as the other main organs inside the body, such as the heart, liver and kidneys. The condition of the gut not only has an effect on your digestive system, but can also impact the ageing process, your immune system, your brain function and your mood. Conditions such as acne, autism, asthma, gastric ulcers, obesity and autoimmune diseases have been closely associated with microbiome and gut health.

DOES IT MATTER WHAT TIME WE EAT?

Sometimes when we eat can be just as important as what we eat. Studies have shown that shortening the time between breakfast and dinner, and lengthening the fast in between dinner and breakfast, can potentially reduce blood sugar, cholesterol and fat. This is because we are increasing the fasting period when we are burning fat. So eating breakfast slightly later and eating dinner slightly earlier can help with maintaining a healthy weight. However, more research needs to be done on this to know exactly how big the difference can be and what more wide-ranging results would show.

Gut bacteria is a big player in how strong the immune system is and how protected you are from diseases such as colitis, Crohn's disease, obesity and even diabetes, and can help with everyday symptoms such as bloating and constipation. Introducing good gut foods from a prebiotic, plant-based diet, including whole grains, fruits, vegetables, nuts and pulses, which help fertilise our existing gut bacteria, and probiotics in food such as fermented food and yoghurts and cheeses, which contain live bacteria, can be beneficial for our gut. Good gut bacteria also have an effect on our metabolism and how well we burn off our fats. These bacteria break down the food we eat into enzymes, vitamins and nutrients that we require to stay healthy.

HEALTH HACKS FOR DIARRHOEA

- make sure you're rehydrating yourself with water
- avoid dairy and sugary food products
- avoid sugary drinks, fruit juices and caffeinated beverages
- make sure to eat small meals
- take over-the-counter medication containing loperamide for any discomfort

What's the difference between an allergy and an intolerance?

Allergies tend to be rarer than intolerances and, in some cases, allergies can actually be life-threatening. True allergies will trigger a full immune response, presenting in a number of different ways, such as difficulty breathing, a rash, sickness and vomiting or a swollen tongue, lips or throat. You should seek urgent medical attention if you have any of these symptoms and, if you have a confirmed allergy, you should make sure you always carry an EpiPen with you.

Intolerances usually have to do with the digestive tract, and these patients may present with tummy pain, diarrhoea, vomiting or excessive gas. Often patients with these symptoms suffer from lactose intolerance, irritable bowel syndrome (IBS) or coeliac disease. Usually by avoiding the food triggers the intolerance can be managed.

Maintaining good immunity

The main ways to improve your immune system naturally are techniques that many people are already aware of. Maintaining a healthy diet is very important because a healthy diet is key to a strong immune system. Make sure your diet is balanced with vegetables, fruits, legumes, greens, proteins and healthy fats (see pages 96–118). Exercising regularly is very important too (see pages 153–70)! Physical activity isn't just for building muscles or looking good in your clothes, it also helps to boost your overall circulation, making it easier for immune cells and other fighting molecules to travel throughout your body. Studies have already shown that engaging in as little as 30 minutes of moderate exercise per day can help support a healthy immune system.

Sleep is also very important when it comes to the immune system. Sometimes it doesn't feel like getting your Zzzzzs is an active process; however there are plenty of important benefits that sleep brings to help your immune system (see pages 171–3 for more information on establishing healthy sleep habits). Being run down and not getting enough sleep weakens your immune system and can put you at risk of catching pesky diseases such as common viral infections like the flu or bacterial infections such as chest infections and UTIs.

Natural ways to boost the immune system – such as getting adequate sleep, exercising, having a balanced, healthy diet, maintaining good gut health, keeping hydrated and managing stress – are better than taking immune-boosting supplements, which is generally used in addition to all these different methods. There is no first-hand evidence that supplementation on its own can boost your immune system.

How can I help hay fever symptoms?

Hay fever is a type of inflammation that occurs when the immune system reacts to allergens. It's characterised by a runny and stuffy nose, sneezing and red, itchy or watery eyes. For some people, this is seasonal due to pollen in the air.

When it comes to treating hay fever, the best way is prevention and avoiding the specific allergens. This can mean not having pets, choosing wooden floors over carpets or other dust-catching furniture at home, and keeping the home dry and ventilated. You can even buy anti-allergy covers for your pillows and mattresses. However, over-the-counter medications, such as antihistamines, provide good relief. If your condition is worsening, sometimes your doctor can prescribe steroid medication or other decongestants.

Pneumonia

Pneumonia is when your lungs get inflamed and infected and this can be caused by viruses or bacteria. Both of these are contagious and can be spread from person to person. The main source of transmission is usually breathing in the air particles from someone else. However, an exchange of saliva or any respiratory tract fluid can also spread the disease. You can also spread the virus by touching your nose or mouth or an object and then somebody touching the same object, hence why we promote good hand hygiene. We also suggest not sharing cups, towels or plates or cutlery with anyone else. And you should sneeze and cough into a tissue which should then be disposed of and then wash your hands thoroughly with soap and water and use alcohol gel appropriately. A good preventative form of medicine is vaccination which we recommend for individuals with chronic long-term conditions, babies and people over the age of 55.

Medical myths

VACCINES CAN GIVE YOU THE DISEASE

I've heard this one a lot, especially regarding the vaccines for Covid-19. The vaccine can't actually give you the disease or any type of flu. Most vaccines are made from DNA or mRNA from the pathogen (aka the germ) or a weakened or dead version of it. They can give you symptoms like a low-grade fever so you don't feel well, but you won't actually have the disease itself.

COLD WEATHER AND BEING OUT IN THE RAIN MAKES YOU SICK

This is one that's been told by parents to their kids for many years. However, studies have shown that, though cold weather may make you feel chillier, you're no more likely to get sick being out in bad weather than if you were in normal weather. You get sick due to pathogens – a germ or organism that causes disease – not the actual weather itself.

How long does the flu last?

Well, how long is a piece of string? This is subjective and often depends on your viral load and the strength of your immune system. Many people have mild symptoms for a few days, while others can feel much worse for much longer. That's why, when it comes to viruses, the best way to combat them is to get vaccinated so you get antibodies and your body has the best chance to fight off the germs and get you better faster. It's also important to get good rest and allow your body to fight off infection.

Six ways to beat the common cold + other viruses

1
Make sure you wash your hands regularly and after using the toilet, and sanitise them when you're out and about.

2
Try having some hot soup – this helps by mirroring the body's action of increasing its temperature to fight off the virus, plus it gets some fluid and nutrients into your body, which can be good because often our appetite falls when we're unwell.

3
Get plenty of rest because the more run down you are the less chance your body has of actually fighting off the infection.

4
Good hygiene is definitely the most important point, so if you're about to sneeze or cough, do it into a tissue, catch it and throw it away, either washing or sanitising your hands afterwards.

5
Having a hot bath is good because, like soup, it can help increase the temperature of your body to help fight off the virus. It's also a good way to relax.

6
Drink lots of fluids to stay hydrated otherwise your body won't have the necessary resources and strength to fight off the infection.

DR. EMEKA'S MINUTES THAT MATTER:
The lunchtime slump

These days, many of us work so hard that we can often get burnt out, frustrated or stressed, and sometimes this can happen by lunchtime. Below are some quick facts and health hacks to use during your lunch break to help you feel fresh and keep continuing on your day's journey of success.

KEEP HYDRATED

Good hydration keeps you going. Choose either plain or naturally flavoured water rather than that tempting coffee which can give you a short buzz but leave you dehydrated and energy-zapped later in the day. If you are a busy person and you're out and about, try to carry a bottle of water with you so you can sip from it regularly. If you're working at a desk, make sure you have a glass of water close by.

STRETCH

Sitting around too much may not sound all that bad as essentially you're not doing anything, right? Wrong. Being deskbound can be bad for your health, and long periods of inactivity have been linked with chronic health diseases such as diabetes, heart disease, obesity, high blood pressure and cholesterol, and deep vein thrombosis (DVT). So get up and stretch regularly – simple neck and back stretches can help reduce or ease chronic neck and back pain.

EAT A HEALTHY, BALANCED LUNCH

Try to make sure your lunch includes a tasty variety of foods, containing some fibre for good gut motility and protein to maintain metabolism and boost muscle growth, as well as a portion or two of your five-a-day. This should give you a good hit of nutrients to keep you going throughout the day. Make sure to prepare lunches in advance. This will not only save you time but have you eating a healthier and cheaper lunch as you won't be tempted to buy those unhealthy fast food options or 'meal deals'. Try to avoid snacking – snacks like crisps and chocolate may seem harmless, but those calories add up!

DISTANCE YOUR SCREEN

Too much screen time has been strongly linked with headaches, eye strain, increased anxiety and poor concentration. If you find yourself looking at a screen/monitor for large periods of the day, make sure to take a break from the screen every hour or so and keep hydrated. Also when working, make sure the screen is a comfortable distance from you and the font is large enough to stop you straining your eyes. If you need specific eyewear, such as contacts or glasses, have these available and use them while working.

BE HYGIENIC

It's imperative that you have an organised and clean workstation – this will not only reduce the chance of infection and maintain hygiene, but can improve productivity too!

You don't need to work in a hospital to have good hand hygiene! Out and about and in the workplace many of us should now be equipped with hand gel and soap and water in the bathrooms. Every time we go to the toilet we should be washing our hands using the correct seven-step method and regularly using hand gel with the same method. This is going to reduce your chance of contracting disease and passing on any germs!

TAKE REGULAR BREAKS

Know your limits and take regular breaks if and when you need to, making sure to listen to your body. Try to get some fresh air – a change of environment and fresh air can really help to clear your mind and improve productivity.

EXERCISE

We can get fit, even at our desks, despite how embarrassing it may seem! Trust me, it's worth those confused stares from your colleagues and will be beneficial to your health in the long run. Try spinal rotations by putting your arms across your body with your hands on the opposite shoulder and rotating left and right. Stretch your shoulders by shrugging them or placing one arm across your body. You can also interlock your fingers and stretch both hands as high above your head as possible with your palms facing the ceiling. For your lower body, you can sit on the edge of your chair and stretch one leg while sitting, keeping it straight, and lean forward until you feel a gentle stretch in your hamstring and then change sides for the opposite leg. Even just a short walk at lunch can be beneficial and help to reduce stress. If you feel you may not be able to attempt these exercises for any medical reasons or doing them causes significant pain, consult your doctor.

AVOID TOO MUCH CAFFEINE

It can be exhausting trying to get through a full day of work, especially when you're running on empty, and many of us turn to our good old friend... coffee. But is that cup of Joe any good for us? And if so, just how good can it be, and how do we know when we're drinking too much?

- **Caffeine is a stimulant and so gets the central nervous system going and helps us feel more alert, alive and active, and less drowsy.**
- **However, too much caffeine can cause restlessness, insomnia, palpitations, stomach ache or even tremors (aka the 'coffee shakes'!).**
- **According to studies, we shouldn't be consuming more than 400–450mg a day (about three cups of coffee or five cups of tea).**
- **Drink no more than the recommended amount, especially if you're experiencing any of the symptoms outlined above, having sleep problems or taking supplementation or other stimulants, such as caffeine or workout pills and nicotine.**
- **Remember that caffeine is also found in tea, fizzy drinks, chocolate and even some medications!**

Below are some approximate reference ranges that might help you gauge your caffeine intake:

- **1 mug of filter coffee = 140mg caffeine**
- **1 mug of instant coffee = 100mg caffeine**
- **1 can of energy drink = 80mg caffeine**
- **1 mug of tea = 75mg caffeine**
- **1 small bar of chocolate = 25–50mg caffeine**
- **1 can of cola = 40mg caffeine**

RECIPES

RECIPES

RECIPES

RECIPES

RECIPES

RECIPES

Protein porridge with almonds + berry citrus compote

SERVES 2
🥄 **15 MINS**
♨ **15-20 MINS**

/ VEGAN
/ DAIRY-FREE

A bowl of porridge is a healthy, filling and nutritious way to start your day. Topped with a zingy berry citrus compote, it is bound to get your morning off to a good start! I like to make a couple of days' worth of compote, which I keep in a jar in the fridge, to make busy weekday mornings that little bit easier.

3 satsumas/easy
   peelers, peeled
90g frozen
   berries, plus a few
   extra to serve
2 tsp runny honey
1 tsp chia seeds
   (optional)
130g porridge oats
200g milk of your
   choice
pinch of ground
   cinnamon
2 tbsp almond butter
1 tbsp mixed seeds
1 tbsp almonds,
   roughly chopped

1 / Cut one satsuma into small dice and place in a small saucepan along with the berries and honey. Cook over a medium heat for 5–10 minutes, stirring occasionally, until the berries have softened. Remove from the heat and add the chia seeds (if using). These will help thicken the compote. Set aside while you make the porridge.

2 / Put the oats, milk and 200ml of water in a medium saucepan and bring slowly to the boil over a gentle heat and simmer for 5–10 minutes until creamy. Add cinnamon to taste and ladle the porridge into two bowls. Top each with 1 tablespoon of almond butter and a generous dollop of the raspberry compote.

3 / Slice the remaining two satsumas and add to the porridge before scattering over a few crushed frozen berries, the seeds and chopped almonds. Serve immediately.

4 / Any leftover compote will keep in an airtight container in the fridge for 3–4 days.

/ THIS WILL PROVIDE A GOOD AMOUNT OF FIBRE, WHICH IS GREAT FOR GUT MOTILITY, AND CARBS WHICH GIVE YOU ENERGY FOR THE DAY!

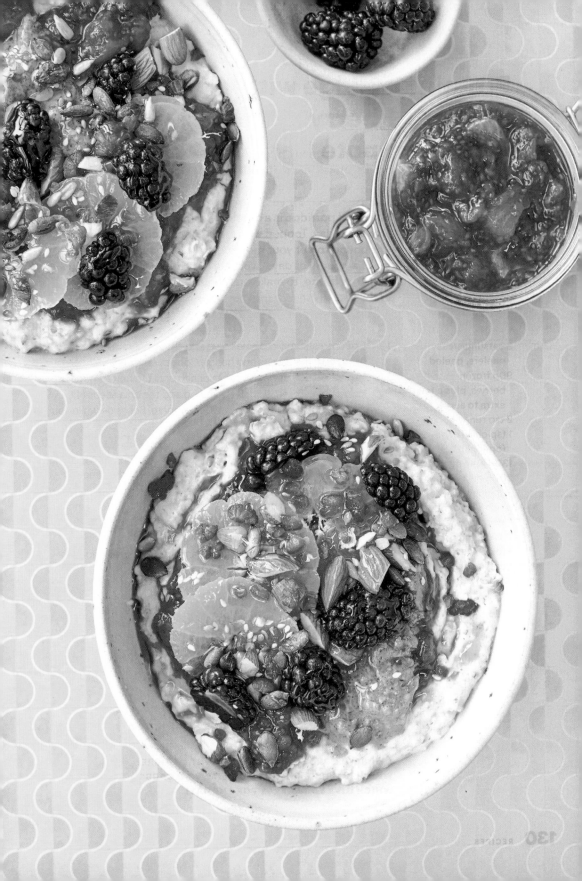

Fruity muesli

SERVES 4
 10 MINS
10 MINS, PLUS COOLING TIME

/ VEGAN
/ DAIRY-FREE

There are so many types of muesli available in the shops now, but I promise you that nothing beats making your own. This recipe is so simple and it is packed with healthy nuts, seeds and dried fruit. Served with milk, berries and a dollop of yoghurt, it makes for a delicious breakfast that will give you a good hit of protein, calcium and fibre, and get you on track towards your five-a-day.

160g jumbo rolled oats
50g pecans, roughly chopped
30g sunflower seeds
30g pumpkin seeds
pinch of ground cinnamon
50g dried cranberries, roughly chopped
50g dried apricots, roughly chopped
100ml milk of your choice
40g yoghurt of your choice
320g mixed fresh berries

1 / Place the oats, pecans, sunflower seeds and pumpkin seeds in a large frying pan and toast over a medium heat for 5–10 minutes, stirring continuously, until the oats are golden. Transfer to a large bowl and leave to cool completely before stirring through the cinnamon, dried cranberries and apricots.

2 / Transfer into four small bowls, pour over the milk and top with Greek yoghurt and fresh berries.

3 / Any remaining muesli will keep in an airtight container for up to 2 weeks.

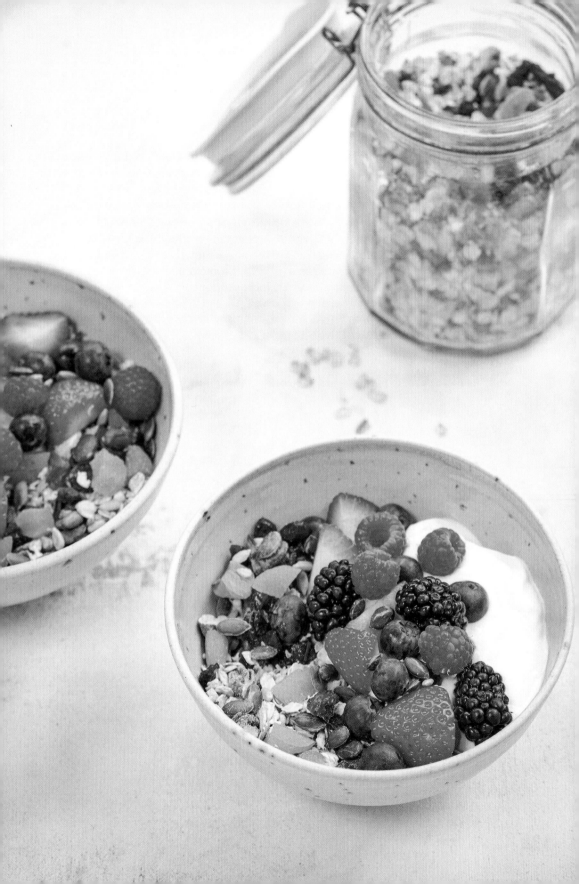

Chocolate protein pancakes with banana + blueberries

SERVES 2
◇ **10 MINS**
♨ **15–20 MINS**

/ VEGETARIAN
/ DAIRY-FREE

Protein is vital for building muscle and is an essential nutrient for the body in terms of recovery. These chocolate protein pancakes are the perfect post-workout breakfast. Topped with fresh fruit, a little syrup and potassium-rich cacao nibs, they also feel decadent enough to make a great weekend brunch treat. I like to add a scoop of protein powder to this recipe, but if you prefer not to then simply replace it with an extra 25g of oats.

FOR THE PANCAKES
1 medium banana
50g porridge oats
25g chocolate, vanilla or plain protein powder (optional)
1 tbsp dark cocoa powder
2 large eggs
30ml milk of your choice
½ tbsp baking powder
1 tbsp smooth peanut butter
1 tsp coconut oil, for frying

TO SERVE
1 banana, thinly sliced
handful of blueberries
2 tbsp cacao nibs
4 tbsp agave syrup, maple syrup or runny honey

1 / Pre-heat the oven to 110°C/90°C fan/gas ¼.

2 / To make the pancakes, place all the ingredients, except the coconut oil, in a blender and blitz until smooth.

3 / Heat half the coconut oil in a large, non-stick frying pan over a medium heat. Ladle spoonfuls of the pancake batter into the pan to make 2–3 round pancakes, being sure to leave space for them to spread slightly. Immediately lower the temperature and cook the pancakes gently for 2–3 minutes or until bubbles appear on the surface. Gently flip each pancake and cook for a further minute before transferring to the warm oven. Repeat with the remaining batter.

4 / To serve, stack the pancakes and top with sliced banana, blueberries and a scattering of cacao nibs. Drizzle with syrup or honey and serve immediately.

/ A DELICIOUS BREAKFAST TO FILL YOU UP AND HELP YOU NATURALLY SUPPORT MUSCLE GROWTH.

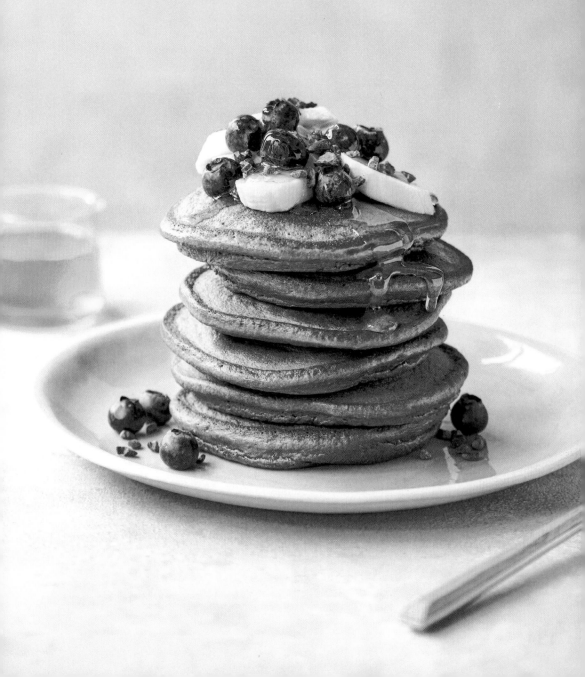

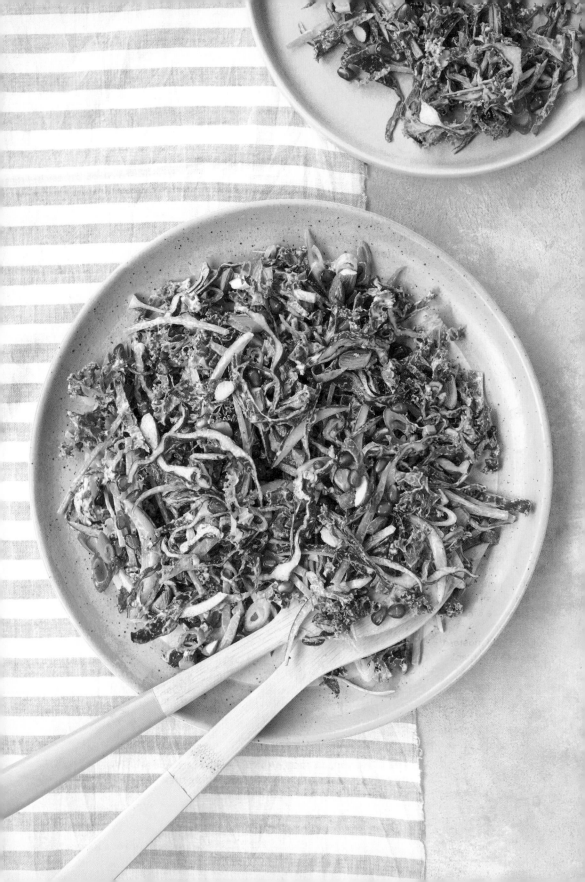

Healthy rainbow coleslaw

SERVES 4
15–20 MINS

/ VEGETARIAN
/ GLUTEN-FREE

Since I was a small child, I have always loved coleslaw. There is nothing like a big bowl of it to go with grilled meat, seafood or veggie burgers. Eating lots of different coloured fruit and vegetables is a great way to help get a wide range of vitamins and minerals into your diet. Keep a batch of this coleslaw in the fridge for easy lunches or make a big, beautiful bowl of it next time you have a barbecue!

½ small red onion, thinly sliced
juice of ½ lime
50g kale, thick stalks removed, leaves finely shredded
½ small red cabbage, core removed, leaves shredded
1 carrot, peeled and cut into thin matchsticks or grated
1 spring onion, finely sliced
2 tbsp low-fat Greek yoghurt
2 tbsp light mayonnaise
2 tsp white wine vinegar
1 tsp Dijon mustard
sea salt and black pepper
50g almonds, roughly chopped, to garnish
2 tbsp pomegranate seeds, to garnish

1 / Place the red onion in a small bowl. Squeeze over the lime juice, mix well and set aside.

2 / Place the kale, red cabbage, carrot and spring onion in a large mixing bowl.

3 / In a separate small bowl, whisk together the Greek yoghurt, mayonnaise, white wine vinegar and Dijon mustard. Season to taste.

4 / Add the dressing to the bowl of vegetables and mix thoroughly so the dressing is evenly distributed.

5 / Transfer the coleslaw to a serving dish and scatter over the almonds and pomegranate seeds. The coleslaw will keep in the fridge for 3–4 days.

/ THE ALMONDS, CARROT AND ONIONS HELP YOU GET YOUR FIVE-A-DAY AND THIS IS A TASTY SIDE DISH BIG IN ENERGY AND LOW IN SALT AND FATS.

Protein noodle stir-fry

SERVES 2
⌀ **15–20 MINS**
♨ **10 MINS**

/ VEGETARIAN
/ DAIRY-FREE

When you need a super-quick, healthy meal, there is nothing like a stir-fry! Many supermarkets now stock delicious, fresh protein noodles made with pea protein or lentils. These are a fantastic substitute for traditional egg noodles and give you that nutritious protein recovery after a workout. For extra protein, you could also add some cooked chicken, cooked prawns or diced tofu.

1 tbsp hoisin sauce
1 tbsp light soy sauce
½ tbsp dark soy sauce
2 tbsp toasted sesame oil
1 large garlic clove, crushed
½ small red chilli, finely chopped
2cm fresh root ginger, peeled and finely chopped
½ red pepper, core removed and finely sliced
100g sugar snap peas
80g broccoli florets, sliced
2 baby pak choi, sliced
275g fresh protein noodles
1 tsp chilli flakes
2 spring onions, finely sliced

1 / In a small bowl, make the sauce by mixing together the hoisin sauce, light and dark soy sauce and 1 tablespoon of the sesame oil. Set aside.

2 / Heat the remaining tablespoon of sesame oil in a large wok or sauté pan over a high heat. Add the garlic, chilli and ginger. Stir-fry for 20–30 seconds until the garlic is fragrant and just starting to colour. Be careful not to let it burn.

3 / Quickly toss in the red pepper, sugar snap peas and broccoli. Stir-fry for 2–3 minutes.

4 / Add the pak choi and continue to fry for 1 minute before adding the noodles, sauce and 50ml of water. Toss everything together and continue to stir-fry for 3–4 minutes until the noodles and vegetables are just cooked and everything is evenly coated in sauce.

5 / Sprinkle over the chilli flakes and spring onions and serve immediately.

/ THIS MEAL IS PACKED WITH PROTEIN, WHICH IS A VERY GOOD MACRONUTRIENT FOR BUILDING STRENGTH.

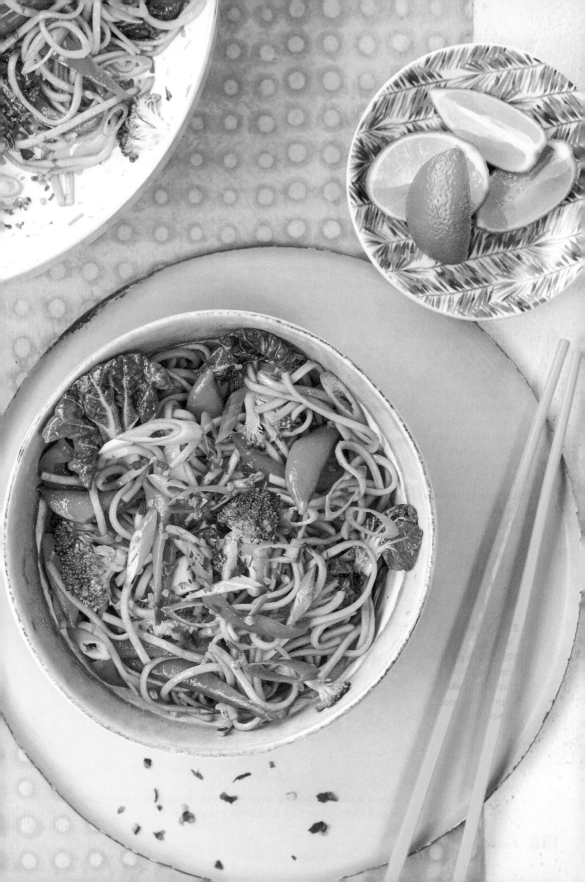

Cod with chorizo, beans + leafy greens

SERVES 2
🥄 **10 MINS**
🍲 **15–20 MINS**

/ GLUTEN-FREE

Fish is a fantastic source of healthy, high-quality protein. I like to grill or bake fish for nutritious, speedy meals that are ready in no time. Paired with smoky chorizo, cannellini beans and lots of leafy greens, this cod dish is an ideal healthy lunch. If you prefer, the cod can be substituted for any other meaty, white fish; hake, haddock or pollock make particularly good alternatives.

1½ tbsp olive oil, plus extra for oiling
100g cooking chorizo, diced
1 large garlic clove, crushed
pinch of chilli flakes
½ tsp ground cumin
½ tsp smoked paprika
1 x 400g can of cannellini beans, drained and rinsed
120g leafy greens (cavolo nero, kale or green cabbage), woody stems removed and leaves chopped
2 x skinless cod fillets, about 120g each
sea salt and black pepper
lemon wedges, to serve

1 / Heat ½ tablespoon of the olive oil in a large frying pan over a medium heat. Add the chorizo and fry for 1–2 minutes.

2 / Add the garlic, chilli flakes, cumin and paprika and fry for 30 seconds, stirring continuously, until the garlic is fragrant.

3 / Pour in the beans and stir together to coat them well in the spices and oil from the chorizo.

4 / Throw in the greens and add a splash of water to help them steam. Toss everything together and continue to cook for 3–4 minutes until the greens are cooked and the beans are warmed through. Season well and set aside.

5 / Heat the grill to the highest setting and oil a baking tray. Place the cod fillets on the oiled tray, drizzle over the remaining olive oil and season well. Grill for 5–8 minutes or until the fish is just cooked.

6 / Transfer the beans and greens to a plate and top with the cod. Squeeze over a lemon wedge before serving.

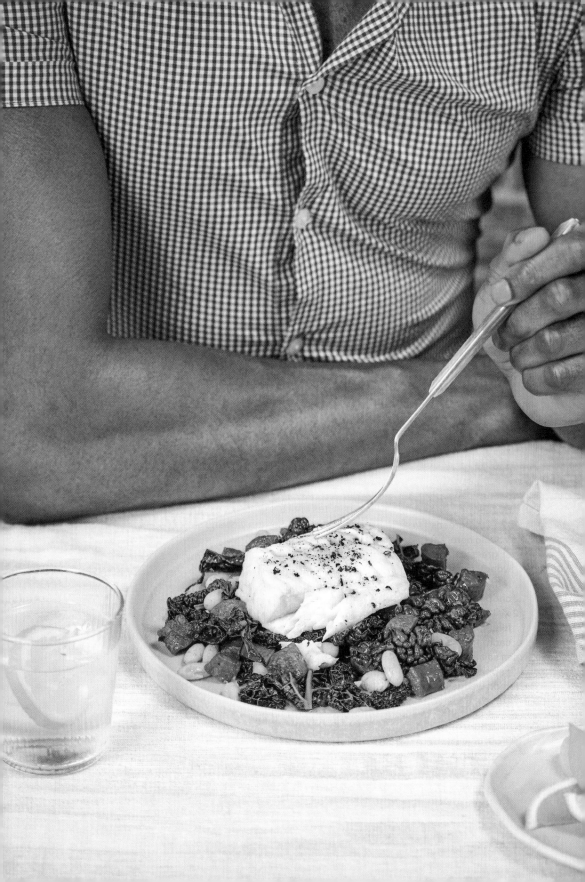

Prawn, edamame + avocado salad

SERVES 4
10-15 MINS

/ GLUTEN-FREE

This beautiful, zingy salad is full of punchy Asian flavours and plenty of protein and vitamins. To make it into a more substantial meal, I sometimes double the amount of dressing and toss through some cooked rice vermicelli noodles. If you are using frozen edamame beans, cook them in boiling, salted water for 3 minutes, drain and rinse in very cold water before adding to the salad.

2 tbsp toasted sesame oil

4 tbsp sweet chilli sauce

2 tsp light soy sauce

zest and juice of 2 limes, plus extra lime wedges to serve

300g king prawns, cooked and peeled

200g edamame beans

1 medium cucumber, deseeded and shaved into ribbons with a vegetable peeler

4 large handfuls of baby leaf salad

2 ripe avocados, stoned, peeled and chopped

2 spring onions, thinly sliced

3 tbsp very roughly chopped coriander, to garnish

2 tbsp mint leaves, to garnish

1 / In a medium bowl, make the dressing by whisking together the sesame oil, sweet chilli sauce, soy sauce, lime zest and juice. Add the prawns to the bowl and toss to coat well in the dressing. Set aside while you make the salad.

2 / In a large mixing bowl, combine the edamame beans, cucumber, salad leaves, avocado and spring onion.

3 / Transfer the salad to a large serving platter, top with the prawns and drizzle over the dressing. Finish by scattering over the coriander and mint leaves.

/ AVOCADOS ARE VERY NUTRITIOUS AS THEY'RE PACKED WITH POTASSIUM WHICH HELPS THE BODY'S CELLS AND NERVES, AND HIGH IN GOOD HEALTHY FATS WHICH CAN COMBAT HEART DISEASE AND STROKE.

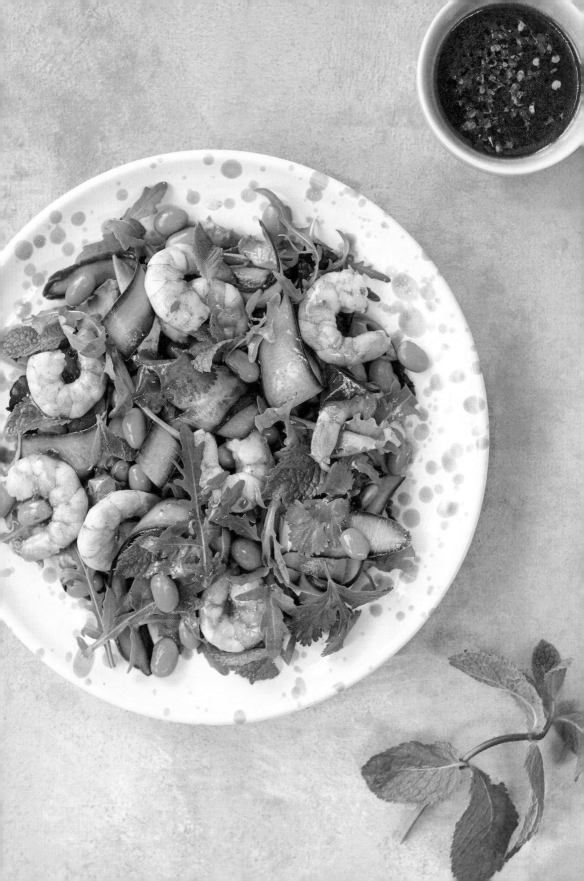

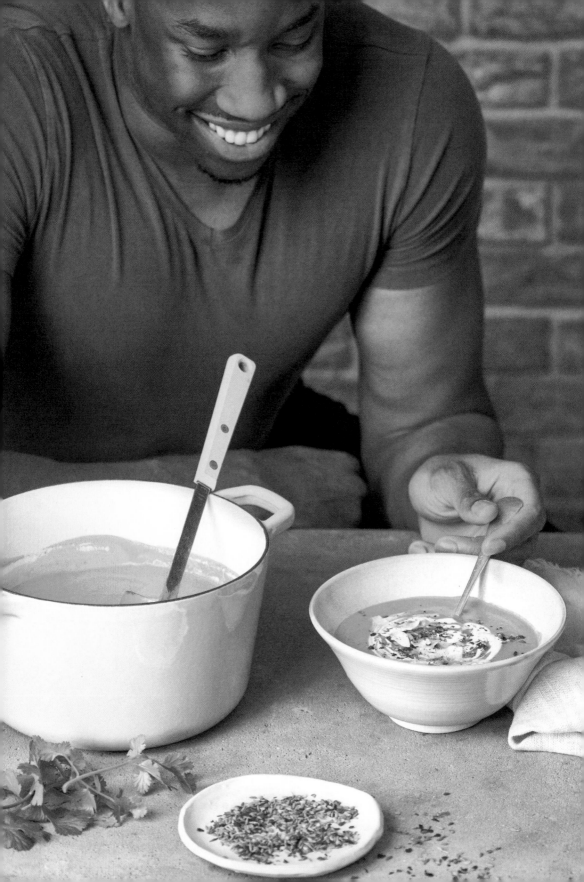

Spiced carrot + red lentil soup

SERVES 4

🍳 **10–15 MINS**

🍲 **20–25 MINS**

/ VEGETARIAN
/ VEGAN
/ GLUTEN-FREE

Lentils are a fantastic, budget-friendly source of fibre, iron and protein. They also count towards one portion of your five-a-day. In this recipe they are teamed with carrots, which are rich in vitamin A, to make a warming, spiced soup laced with coconut milk. It is a perfect recipe to make a big batch of for convenient mealtimes. It keeps in an airtight container in the fridge for 3–4 days, or freeze individual portions for whenever you need a quick, nutritious meal!

1 tbsp coconut oil
100g onion, diced
1 large garlic clove, grated
500g carrots, peeled and diced
1 tsp ground turmeric
1 tsp ground cumin
½ tsp mild curry powder
150g split red lentils
800ml hot vegetable stock
125ml coconut milk, plus extra to serve
sea salt and black pepper
2 tbsp coconut chips (optional), to garnish
½ tbsp cumin seeds, toasted, to garnish
1 tsp chilli flakes, to garnish
a few coriander leaves, to garnish

1 / Heat the coconut oil in a large, heavy-based saucepan over a medium heat and add the onion, garlic and carrot. Allow the vegetables to sweat for 5 minutes, stirring often.

2 / Add the spices and season well. Mix well and continue to cook for 2 minutes.

3 / Add the lentils to the pan, stir together and pour over the vegetable stock and coconut milk. Bring to a gentle simmer and cook for 15 minutes or until both the lentils and carrots are soft.

4 / Transfer the soup to a blender and blitz until smooth. Check the seasoning before ladling the soup into four bowls. Drizzle with a little coconut milk and scatter over the coconut chips (if using), cumin seeds, chilli flakes and a few coriander leaves.

/ VITAMIN A IS GREAT FOR SUPPORTING EYE HEALTH.

Chicken satay salad

SERVES 2

🥘 15 MINS, PLUS
   MARINATING TIME

🍲 15-20 MINS

/ GLUTEN-FREE

Spiced chargrilled chicken, creamy peanut sauce and fresh, crisp salad is a winning combination. Big on protein and flavour, it is exactly what you need for your last meal of the day. The sauce is also brilliant for dipping raw vegetables in as a healthy snack.

2 x boneless skinless chicken breasts, about 175g each

1 large garlic clove, crushed

1 tsp runny honey

1 tsp ground turmeric

1 tsp mild curry powder

1 tsp tamari

2 tsp vegetable oil

2 baby gem lettuce, leaves separated and washed

½ red onion, thinly sliced

small bunch of coriander

½ small cucumber, diced

1 lime, cut into wedges, to serve

FOR THE SATAY SAUCE

80ml coconut milk

2 tbsp crunchy peanut butter

1 tbsp fresh lime juice

½ tbsp mild curry powder

½ tbsp tamari

½ tbsp runny honey

½ tsp lemongrass paste (optional)

1 / Place one chicken breast between two sheets of parchment paper and gently bash with a rolling pin or meat tenderiser to flatten it to a uniform thickness of about 1.5–2cm. This will help the chicken cook evenly. Repeat with the second chicken breast.

2 / In a large bowl or Tupperware, combine the garlic, honey, turmeric, curry powder, tamari and 1 teaspoon of the vegetable oil along with 2 tablespoons of cold water to make a loose paste. Add the chicken breasts and coat them well in the mix. Cover and leave to marinate in the fridge for a minimum of 2 hours or preferably overnight.

3 / To make the sauce, combine all the ingredients in a small pan over a low heat. Bring to a boil and simmer for 3–5 minutes until it has thickened to a pourable sauce.

4 / When you are ready to eat, heat a griddle pan over a high heat until very hot. Remove the chicken breasts from the marinade, scraping off the excess with a spoon. Brush the chicken with the remaining vegetable oil and grill for 5–6 minutes per side or until it is cooked through. Remove from the heat and leave to rest while you finish the salad.

5 / On a large serving platter, arrange the baby gem leaves and scatter over the red onion, coriander and cucumber.

6 / Slice the chicken breast into 1cm slices and arrange on the salad. Drizzle over the satay sauce and serve with wedges of lime.

/ THIS SALAD IS EASY TO PREPARE, SIMPLE TO COOK AND PACKED WITH ESSENTIAL VITAMINS AND MINERALS.

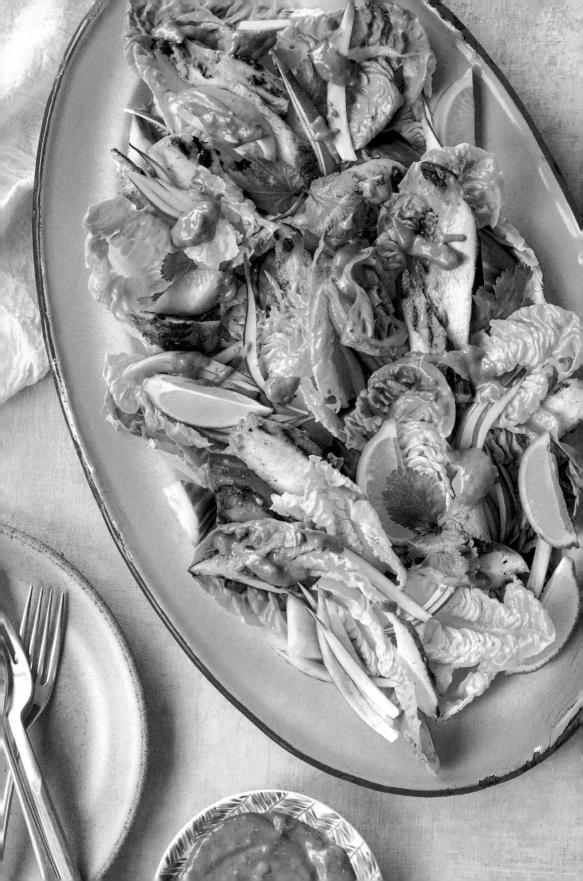

Baked eggs in a quick tomato sauce

SERVES 4
🥄 **5–10 MINS**
🍲 **20–25 MINS**

/ VEGETARIAN
/ GLUTEN-FREE

This dish is so quick and easy to put together. Serve it with some crusty bread and you have a nourishing and tasty meal that is perfect for everything from a speedy weeknight dinner to a leisurely weekend brunch. I sometimes add chopped ham, chorizo or some cannellini beans to the sauce for a bit of extra protein.

200g baby leaf
  spinach
1 tbsp olive oil
1 large garlic clove,
  crushed
½ tsp chilli flakes
1 tsp ground cumin
¼ tsp ground allspice
1 x 400g can of
  good-quality
  chopped tomatoes
1 tsp balsamic
  vinegar
4 medium eggs
sea salt and black
  pepper

1 / Pre-heat the oven to 200°C/180°C fan/gas 6.

2 / Place the spinach in a colander and pour over a kettle of freshly boiled water to wilt the leaves. Run cold water over the spinach to stop it cooking. Squeeze out any excess water and set aside.

3 / Heat the olive oil in a medium saucepan over a medium heat. Add the garlic and chilli and fry for 15 seconds. Add the spices and stir well for another 10–15 seconds or until fragrant.

4 / Pour in the tomatoes and stir well before adding the balsamic vinegar and some seasoning. Bring the tomato sauce to the boil and simmer for 10 minutes until it is thick and rich.

5 / Divide the tomato sauce between four small ovenproof dishes. Scatter over the cooked spinach.

6 / Use a spoon to make a small well in the middle of the tomato sauce in each dish and crack an egg into the well. Sprinkle the egg with sea salt and black pepper.

7 / Bake in the oven for 12–15 minutes or until the egg white is just set and the yolk still a little runny.

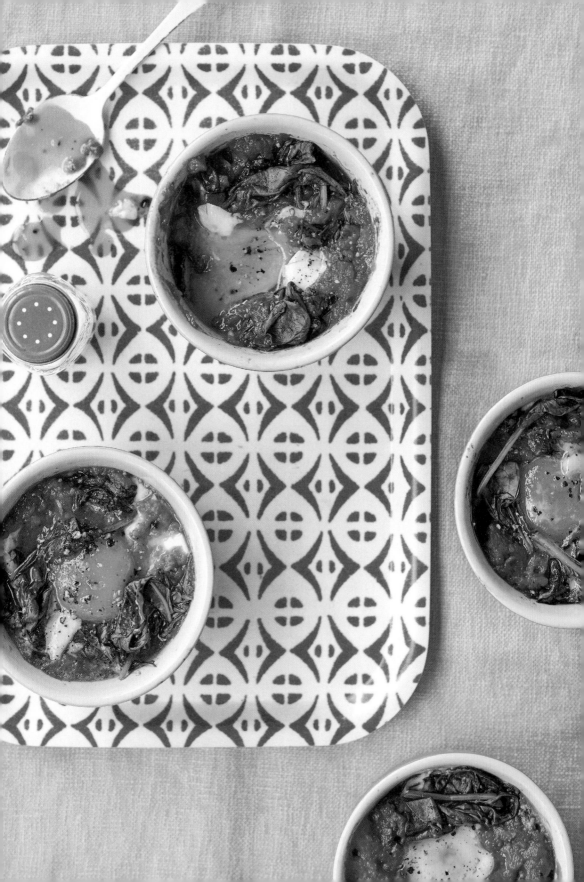

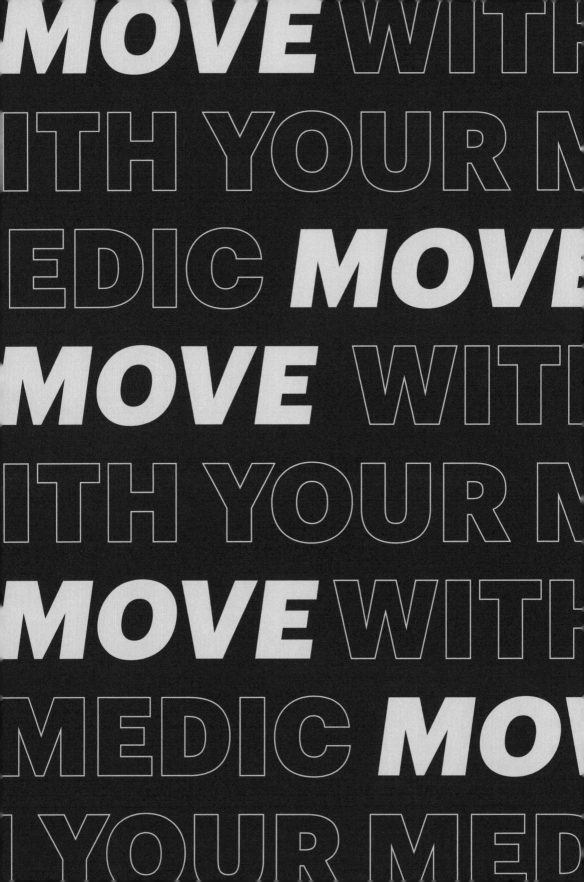

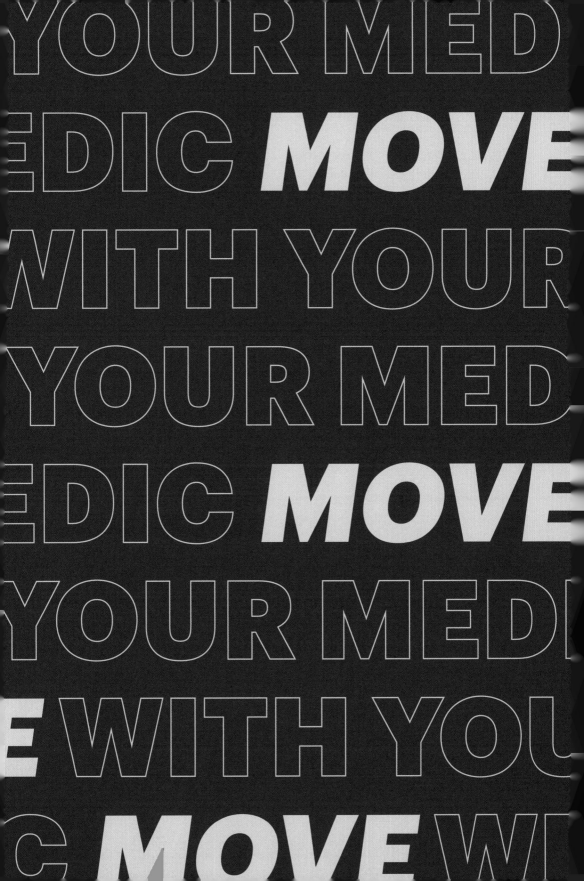

THE BENEFITS OF BEING ACTIVE

MOTIVATION

Sometimes it can be hard to get ourselves motivated to make the best of our day. When this happens, I tend to turn to what gets me in the best mental and physical state. To psych myself up for a good day, depending on my work schedule, I listen to podcasts and books, and make sure to get an early run or workout session in.

I'm a huge advocate for fitness, health and keeping the body in optimum shape. Throughout my life, whether through team or individual sports, I've always seen how important exercise can be, both physically and mentally. I think it's imperative to show my patients that I'm physically fit, exercise regularly and take my health seriously, so as to encourage them to do the same. If I come in to see a patient looking healthy and physically athletic from exercising, it hopefully encourages them to follow in my footsteps, and thus they can improve their own health too.

However, when I qualified as a doctor, I soon learnt that keeping up with fitness and sports while juggling a busy, demanding job was a very difficult task. Due to the nature of the job, often I wouldn't leave until hours after my shift had finished, as tasks needed to be completed before it was safe for me to leave my patients.

And for the first time since I could remember, I wasn't able to go to training or play any sports, and the impact on my physical and mental health was evident. I felt isolated and alone; I felt overworked and unhealthy. At one point, the burnout became unbearable and I knew something needed to change. I wasn't my happy, healthy self anymore. I was unfit, unhappy and unable to cope. And so I made a regime for home workouts. I started making my own healthy, nutritious meals and I cut out the takeaways and fast foods I was constantly buying, due to both lack of time and laziness, and instead cooked tasty, nutritious meals. As a result, I slowly started to see my old self coming back.

It was evident that my mental health, which was now improved, was closely linked to how well I was eating and how often I was exercising. Not only does exercise benefit you in the long term by preventing chronic disease, but in the short term it can help boost your mood and can give you an emotional lift, which will help you blow off some steam after a long day, which is often the case with me and my work.

Any kind of physical activity can stimulate various brain chemicals such as endorphins and leave you feeling happier, more relaxed and less anxious. I really believe that looking good and feeling good go hand-in-hand, and exercise encompasses this theory completely. But more on the importance of good mental health in the next section (pages 174–93)!

Engaging in regular physical activity and burning calories is one of the best ways to keep yourself healthy, and the benefits of exercise are almost endless from a medical point of view. We know how well exercise helps control weight; it can help prevent excess weight gain and maintain weight loss. Strength training and cardiovascular exercise can also be great for muscle building. Working in the NHS, I can see that many of the conditions people present with in A&E or diseases that I've seen working in GP practices – such as stroke, metabolic syndrome, high blood pressure, diabetes, anxiety, depression, many types of cancer and heart disease – can all be helped by regular exercise.

Another really important reason I exercise is for the energy boost. Everything I do in terms of medical and media work needs energy, whether that is seeing patients or trying to engage people on social media. Exercise delivers oxygen and nutrients to your tissues and helps your cardiovascular system work more efficiently. When your heart and lung health improves, you have more energy to tackle daily chores – and it helps me to make a lot of entertaining videos too! It's pretty obvious that there are so many benefits to exercise and yet I find it baffling that some people simply refuse to exercise, or find an excuse as to why they shouldn't. I hope my easy tips and hacks in this section will inspire you to get that blood pumping!

Medical myth

YOU SHOULD WAIT AN HOUR AFTER EATING BEFORE YOU GO SWIMMING

This is a rumour that comes from the fact that vigorous exercise after eating can be quite uncomfortable. But there's no proof that swimming poses any harm after having a meal.

The ten benefits of regular exercise

1 IT HELPS TO REDUCE CHRONIC PAIN

2 IT CAN MAKE YOU FEEL HAPPIER

3 IT STIMULATES WEIGHT LOSS

4 IT INCREASES MUSCLE AND BONE DENSITY

5 IT IMPROVES FATIGUE + INCREASES ENERGY

6 IT REDUCES RISK FACTORS FOR CHRONIC DISEASES LIKE CANCER, HEART DISEASE + DIABETES

7 IT HELPS IMPROVE SLEEP QUALITY

8 IT HELPS WITH ANTIOXIDANTS, KEEPING YOUR SKIN YOUNG AND HEALTHY

9 IT INCREASES YOUR LIFE SPAN – SO LIVE LONG AND PROSPER!

10 IT HELPS WITH BRAIN FUNCTION + MEMORY

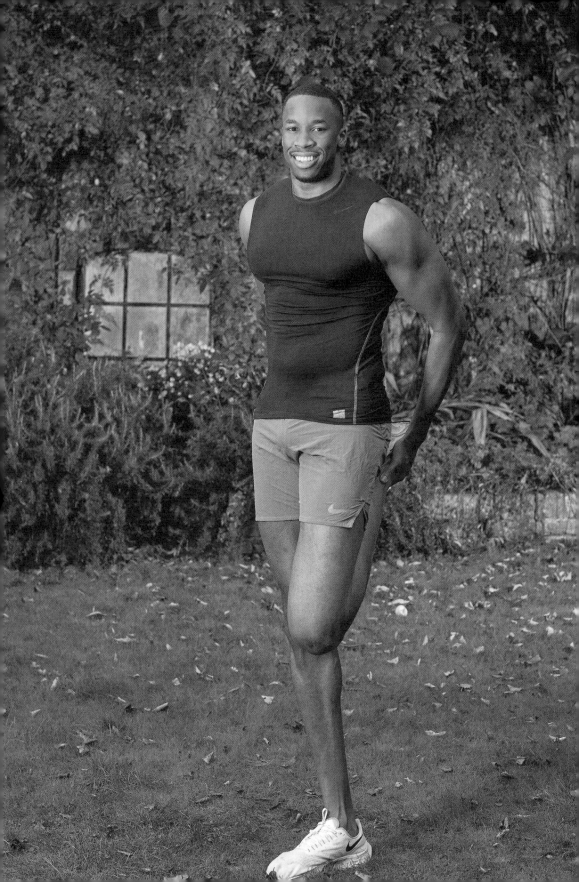

A&E STORY

A 42-year-old gentleman came into A&E as he had been
suffering with sharp chest pains for a few weeks. He said
they were getting much worse when he was walking around
his house or going to work. Exertional chest pains are a
sign of what we call ischaemia. This means that the blood
circulation to the heart and muscle isn't optimal. In the UK
ischaemic heart disease is one of the biggest killers.

I spoke to the gentleman about his lifestyle choices. He
admitted he wasn't living a very healthy lifestyle, often
eating fast food on the road and he hadn't exercised in
years. He claimed it was mainly because of his job as a lorry
driver and that he didn't have the time. He also admitted
that he smoked a few packs of cigarettes daily and often
drank excessively when he wasn't working. I warned him
about the dangers of his lifestyle and what it could lead to.
Unfortunately, I was sad to hear after we treated and started
him on the relevant medications that he suffered a heart
attack and cardiac arrest a few months later and passed
away. This was very difficult for me to process because
I couldn't be sure whether or not he had listened to my
advice and changed his lifestyle and unfortunately still
passed away or if he just went back to his old ways and his
death could have been prevented. Either way, it highlights
how serious the effects of poor lifestyle habits and choices
can be, and how much they can impact our health.

EASY WAYS TO ADD MOVEMENT INTO YOUR DAY

MOTIVATION

When the journey gets rough, never forget that the harder you've worked for something, the greater you'll feel when you get it. When you feel like quitting, just remember why you started.

To be strong and at your optimum physically is one of the greatest things you can do for your health. And it's no surprise that this comes from regular exercise and keeping your body moving. Living a sedentary lifestyle can lead to some serious physical health risks which could eventually slow down your metabolism, weaken your muscles, cause you to gain weight and increase your bad cholesterol and even your blood sugars. And this essentially will shorten your lifespan. On the other hand, building regular exercise routines that you're doing every day will prove to be particularly beneficial and extend your lifespan by reducing the risk of cardiovascular disease.

What exactly is exercise?

Exercise is any movement requiring your body to work and burn calories. This could include lifting weights, running, swimming or – one of my favourites – dancing! Research suggests that at least 150 minutes a week of moderate aerobic activity or 75 minutes a week of vigorous aerobic activity, or a combination of the two, can help the cardiovascular system and prevent disease. Examples include running, walking or swimming. Strength-training exercises for major muscle groups at least two times a week have been known to be very beneficial for your health. Good examples include lifting free weights, using weight machines, doing bodyweight training, climbing stairs and doing yoga or Pilates.

Maintenance is super important as well. Your bones, muscles and joints all want to work together to make your body a mobile machine. Like any other machine, your body can suffer from wear and tear and it needs regular maintenance. This means physical self-care such as stretching and recovery. Building healthy habits of stretching before and after a workout and making sure you allow for regular recovery is just as important as going to the gym. Taking time to stretch and warm up will help prevent any injuries and actually improve the efficacy of the workout.

Find the exercise that's right for you

There are a number of different exercises encompassing cardio, toning, core, stretching and warming up. It's helpful to have a good bank of exercises so you can mix up your workouts and keep your enthusiasm throughout the week. This could include dancing, rollerblading, skating, Zumba, yoga, skipping, cycling or gymnastics.

The key is consistency and to spread the activities throughout the week to make sure you're doing different things every day depending on your fitness goals. And if this is something you enjoy, you're far more likely to stick to it. Exercise is fun, it's free and the positive effects it has on your mental and physical health are staggering.

Medical myth

IF YOU'RE EXERCISING AND NOT LOSING WEIGHT, YOU'RE DOING SOMETHING WRONG

This isn't always the case. Yes, when you exercise well enough and you're using more calories than you consume, you're likely to lose weight. However, you can be exercising in a way that you're gaining muscle mass and muscle actually weighs more than fat. So you may be getting in better shape, but your actual defined weight may not change that much.

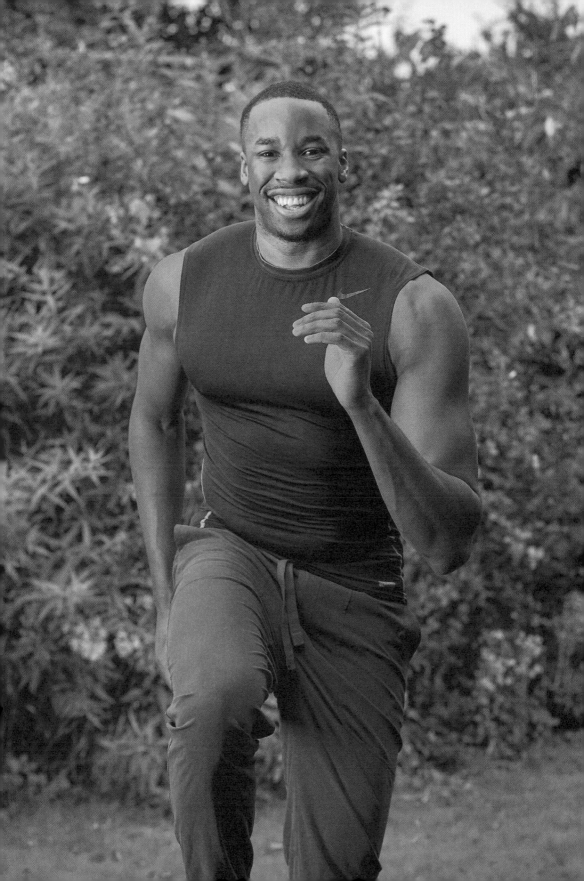

How to get fit in your own home

Your home may be your comfort zone, but with many of us working from home more regularly since the beginning of the coronavirus pandemic or not having the time or inclination to go to the gym, we've all had to adapt and learn how to get fit at home.

My motto has always been 'no gym, no problem'! As long as you're getting the five elements of a good fitness programme done, you'll be getting a good workout:

1. **A warm up**
2. **A cardiovascular workout of some sort**
3. **A resistance and strength-building workout**
4. **A flexibility and stretching session**
5. **A cool down**

If you're a beginner, try to aim for about 30 minutes of cardio and 20–30 minutes of strength training at least 3 times a week, and build up once you feel more confident.

A FEW TIPS TO HELP KEEP YOU GOING INCLUDE:

- **Challenge yourself and avoid boredom. Try to mix up the exercises every day.**
- **Find an exercise partner who you can workout at home with. You'll be less likely to make excuses with that kind of accountability.**
- **Schedule your workouts so you have some sort of plan and organisation – use a planner if you need to.**
- **Try to track your progress via an app or journal so you can see that you're gradually getting better over time.**
- **Set some goals, such as getting ready for a marathon or being able to do a particular number of reps by a certain date.**
- **If you need to, give yourself some rewards along the way to give you that extra little bit of motivation.**

If you have any questions about your abilities and what your medical conditions will allow you to do safely, make sure you speak to a doctor for medical advice. Normally most moderate exercise is safe for the majority of people. However, in certain circumstances, a number of people can only do specific moves. This is different for everybody, so if you are in any doubt, make sure you check with your doctor before starting a new exercise regime.

Three tips to get back into exercise

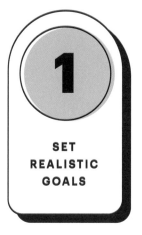

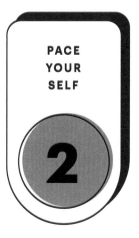

Why train outside?

Come rain or shine, there is no excuse not to take your training outside. Fresh air is not only a great boost for your motivation and general mental well-being, but the physical benefits of training outside can have an amazing effect on the release of so-called 'happiness hormones', like oxytocin, endorphins and dopamine (see opposite).

Taking your training outside can even boost your immune system. Getting out of the house can be good for your mood, and a change of environment can be really beneficial to reduce stress and take your mind off work, especially if you're working from home. Try some group exercises or simply go for a run. It doesn't matter what you do, as long as you get up, get out and go get fit!

CHEAT WAYS TO GET STRONGER

- **Make the exercises work for you – if this means doing them at home on a chair for convenience, then do it.**
- **Plan your day around your workout times so you have no excuses not to get stuck in!**
- **Make it something enjoyable that you actually take pleasure in. Try listening to an audiobook, podcast or your favourite tunes every time you run to the office, join a group class or catch up on your favourite TV show while working out on the treadmill at the gym.**
- **Use resistance bands and body weights if you can't get to the gym, or get your mitts on some dumbbells or kettlebells – now you have no excuse!**

The four chemicals for happinesss

2

DOPAMINE
(THE REWARD CHEMICAL)

This is stimulated when you do self-care activities; little wins like finding a good parking space, the satisfaction of completing a task or making really good food!

1

SEROTONIN
(THE MOOD STABILISER)

This is stimulated by things like nice walks in nature, meditation and light exercise such as swimming, cycling and jogging.

3

OXYTOCIN
(THE LOVE CHEMICAL)

This one gets stimulated by doing stuff like hugging a baby (they're so cute!) or giving compliments or kisses.

4

ENDORPHINS
(THE NATURAL PAINKILLER)

These are generated by things like working hard and belly laughter.

SO LET'S ALL GET OUTSIDE, GET SOME GOOD EXERCISE AND HAVE FUN WITH THE PEOPLE WE LOVE, DOING WHAT WE LOVE!

SETTING FITNESS GOALS

MOTIVATION

It's not enough to want it to happen, or wish it to happen; you have to get up, go out there and make it happen.

Sometimes people can get overwhelmed by the thought of going to the gym and lifting weights. However, the key is to start off slow, give yourself goals and build up gradually. Sometimes when it's too overwhelming people tend to quit. Perhaps you could start by focusing on losing a couple of kg over a few weeks, or improving your 'one rep max' for a compound lift, or improving your time for a 5k run. That way you can aim to get better and better every day, every week, every month. Soon you'll see big differences from small changes. The way to stay strong physically is to be enthusiastic about it, so make sure you're keeping it fun and light. This might also mean changing your routine, sometimes working out with friends, and you can even try taking up a new sport.

Failure, like many things in life, is an illusion... In this life, you set your goals, you visualise them, you pray for them and then you work for them relentlessly until they become your reality. You may fail – many of us do – but you do have to get back up, you have to keep going forward, you have to push yourself, you have to believe you can do it!

The benefits of exercise only really come with long-term consistency. So it's key to find a good way of challenging yourself every day to make sure that you keep going, and keep progressing.

Medical myth

LIFTING WEIGHTS WILL MAKE YOU LOOK CHUNKY

Many people feel that if they start lifting weights they'll look too pumped up and so are put off by the idea. Though there may be some truth to this, there are certain ways of lifting weights that actually help you to get stronger and strengthen and tone those muscles without necessarily making them much bigger, so don't write it off before you've even given it a go. There are many benefits to strength training and your body will reap the rewards in the long run.

Three tips to motivate yourself

No matter what we're doing, we all want to stay motivated. Being enthusiastic and motivated in any field can improve your mental health and your performance. A lot of people struggle with motivation so I've come up with three tips to help you to keep going:

1. **Reward yourself when you achieve your goals. Set little goals and make sure that when you get them, you give yourself a small reward. This could be seeing a family member or friend you haven't seen in a while or doing an activity you love that you don't normally get time for.**

2. **Find somebody in your field, someone close to you or someone else who you really admire and use that and their achievements as motivation for you. My mother and father have been grinding for years in their respective fields while raising me and my siblings. To see them do all that and achieve success is all the motivation I need. No matter where I go or what I do, I owe everything to my parents.**

3. **Always refer to your baseline. Anything we do has a reason. So always remember why you started and use that as motivation to power on and do your best.**

How do I get the most out of my workout?

1. **Turn off your phone or TV:** this is going to limit rest and sitting time and you're far less likely to procrastinate.

2. **Work out with a buddy:** find a friend to motivate and push you. Sometimes workouts can be less daunting with a friend. Also, if you work out with a friend, you're far more likely to push yourself to get a PB, especially when lifting weights, as you have someone to spot you.

3. **Spread your workout:** sometimes a long workout can be overwhelming. Try breaking it up over the day. So instead of a 90-minute workout, try 45 minutes in the morning maybe doing cardio and then 45 minutes in the evening doing something different like weights.

How to work out around a busy schedule

Many of us struggle to fit exercise into busy lives. It may be that exercise is the last thing on your mind. And sometimes going to the gym just isn't accessible or available – or even appealing! – to everybody. However, you can exercise anywhere, anyhow, any time...

2 TAKE AN EXERCISE BREAK

If you work from home, take regular breaks from your desk, run up and down the stairs, go for a short walk around the block, run on the spot, walk the kids to school rather than taking the car or try some quick aerobic activities like burpees or squats to get that heart pumping and those muscles firing.

1 TRY TO EXERCISE ON YOUR COMMUTE

If you have to go into the office, try swapping up taking public transport to either run or cycle, or even just walk, to work.

3 SCHEDULE YOUR WORKOUTS LIKE YOU SCHEDULE YOUR MEETINGS

Prioritise them and make sure they're in your calendar and you're reminded about them constantly. Then it's going to be far less likely that you'll forget.

4 GET UP EVEN EARLIER

Be an early bird and try to do your workouts before the kids wake up or your other half goes into the office. This might mean a little bit less sleep, but a little bit more exercise might be more beneficial for your health. However, adequate rest is important for recovery of the body and mind so you might want to get an earlier night to compensate.

5 JOIN A GYM THAT'S CONVENIENT

Sometimes having a gym near the office or near your workspace makes exercise less of a task. If you do shift work and start or finish at crazy o'clock, try to join a gym that's 24 hours so you can go before or after work.

DR. EMEKA'S MINUTES THAT MATTER:

The night-time wind down

Sleep is vital for our overall health and key to a happier, healthier and longer life, but it also allows muscles, organs and the brain to recover and repair each night. It is recommended that we get about 7–8 hours' sleep per night, though this varies from person to person.

A good night's sleep is just as important as regular exercise and a healthy diet. Research shows that poor sleep has a negative effect on your hormones, exercise performance, brain function and mood, so it is important to maintain a healthy circadian rhythm to optimise your health.

The circadian rhythm, the body's clock, is a 24-hour cycle that is part of the body's internal clock, running in the background to carry out essential functions and processes. One of the most important and well-known circadian rhythms is the sleep–wake cycle. Your body's circadian rhythm functions on a set loop aligning itself with sunrise and sunset – regulating cycles of alertness and sleepiness by responding to light changes. Without a properly functioning circadian rhythm, our bodies are prone to exhaustion, mental disorders, obesity and other physical illness. Your circadian rhythm helps you maintain a healthy sleep–wake schedule to function properly. Keeping it in check is important to stay mentally and physically healthy.

Interestingly, the circadian rhythm isn't quite the same for men and women. Women tend to sleep earlier at night than men and are more likely to be early birds. They also need about 20 more minutes of sleep to function at cerebral capacity.

OVERCOMING INSOMNIA

If you're struggling to sleep, try listening to binaural beats on your phone app or even on YouTube. They're an auditory illusion created by your brain when two tones with different frequencies are played separately. Research shows they have the ability to reduce stress and anxiety and thus help combat insomnia. Listening to two beat sounds at slightly different frequencies causes the brain to generate an additional beat which is the difference between the frequencies. This affects brainwave activity, prolonging deep sleep and improving quality of sleep.

THE GOOD NEWS IS THAT THERE ARE SO MANY EASY HACKS WE CAN USE TO OPTIMISE OUR SLEEP:

BE CONSISTENT

One of the best things we can do is to try to go to sleep and wake up at the same times throughout the week. Being consistent with your sleep can help improve sleep quality. Some studies have highlighted that irregular sleep patterns can alter the circadian rhythm and the hormone melatonin which signal your brain to sleep. I know this isn't always easy, and sometimes late nights or early mornings can't be prevented, but if you can, try to make sure you have a consistent sleep and wake time to get a good night's rest.

GET THE LIGHT RIGHT

Increasing bright light exposure during the day and having a very dark room when you're trying to fall asleep has been known to improve sleep quality and reduce the time taken to fall asleep.

Reducing blue light exposure in the evening is imperative to having a good night's sleep; this is because it has an effect on your circadian rhythm, tricking your brain into thinking it's daytime, thus reducing hormones like melatonin which help you relax and get to sleep. You can wear glasses that block blue light or make sure you stop watching TV and turn off any bright lights and devices at least two hours before going to bed.

AVOID CAFFEINE TOO CLOSE TO BEDTIME

Caffeine has a number of benefits – a single dose can help us focus, give us energy and boost sports performance. However, it doesn't help you when it comes to sleeping. When you consume it late in the day, caffeine stimulates the nervous system and stops your body from fully relaxing at night. Caffeine can stay in your blood for about 6–8 hours and studies show that caffeine shouldn't be consumed less than 6 hours before going to bed (see page 127 for more facts about caffeine).

REDUCE REGULAR OR LONG DAYTIME NAPS

While short power naps are beneficial for a number of people, long irregular napping during the day can negatively affect your sleep. If you take regular daytime naps and also sleep well this is fine, however the effects of napping depend on the individual and many people have reported poor night-time sleeping and difficulty getting to sleep at night after taking a daytime nap.

OPTIMISE YOUR BEDROOM ENVIRONMENT

Many people believe that an optimum bedroom environment sets you up for a good night's sleep. Factors include temperature, noise, external lights, furniture arrangement and comfortable bedding. Studies have shown that many people noticed improved sleep quality when noise and light were diminished, so make sure your bedroom is quiet, relaxing and comforting.

FUN FACTS ABOUT SLEEP

- **Apparently, the record for the longest amount of time without sleep is 11 days.**
- **The dreams we have are related to our everyday senses, such as sight, sound, touch and smell.**
- **Ever found it hard to get out of bed in the morning? (Me too!) There's actually a medical name for this – dysania.**
- **Speaking of medical terms, parasomnia is movement during sleep.**
- **Twenty-one per cent of the British population sleeps in the foetal position (not me – I like to spread out!).**

YOUR MIND

MAT

TERS

LOOKING AFTER YOUR MENTAL HEALTH

'

MOTIVATION

Along your journey, there will be doubters, naysayers, people who won't understand your struggle or your destiny. But the only person limiting your greatness is you! People may tell you to walk, talk and look a certain way, but it's time to break the mould, think outside the box, stand out and be noticed! Fear can be your biggest hurdle or your greatest motivator... but today only you can decide.

'

You've gotta look after your mind! Mental health is just as important as physical health, and if your mind isn't working well, then your body won't be working well either. You can be your best doctor when it comes to your mental health. There are so many self-care techniques and lifestyle changes that can help you to improve your mental health, many of which – such as maintaining a healthy diet, introducing exercise into your day and getting a good night's sleep – we've already discussed. Sometimes these little changes can even prevent some mental health problems from developing or getting worse. In this chapter I've shared some simple tips and hacks that I hope will help you in supporting your mental health.

MEDITATE

I love to start my day with some quiet down time. Take a minute out – or even five – to just sit and meditate, whether it's by yourself or listening to soothing sounds or even using an app. This can help reduce stress and anxiety, put you in a relaxed state and support you throughout the day.

KEEP TALKING

We need to make sure our mental health is as optimal as possible because that determines our mood and generally how we feel. One of the best ways to maintain good mental health is making sure you're talking about your feelings. It's not always easy describing how you're feeling, and many of us find it hard, but you need to make sure you have someone or different people you can talk to about how you feel and have the courage to just let it out. If you don't have a massive network of family and friends, then forums and support groups online provided by the NHS or charities like Mind (mind.org.uk) can be very useful.

STAY CONNECTED

Creating strong family ties and friendships is really important for mental health. Supportive friends and family can help us deal with the stresses of life; they can keep us active and grounded and help solve mental and practical problems. For me, my strength, my faith and my belief have been largely due to my amazing parents. They believed in me way back when I barely believed in myself. Through every low point I've had, they've always been the first to support me, and in every successful moment, they have been right there to cheer me on.

As sociable animals, we love to keep up with each other face-to-face, but sometimes that's not possible, so make sure you use your social media or a phone call to keep in touch with people. But be aware of some of the dangers of social media, such as peer pressure and imposter syndrome, and be careful not to compare yourself or your situation to others online (see pages 185–6 for more on the effects of social media and how to engage with it in a healthy way).

KEEP ACTIVE

As we saw in the last section, physical exercise is really beneficial for mental health, in the same way that good mental health benefits how you are physically. The chemicals and neurotransmitters released from exercise are great for your mood. This doesn't always have to mean going to the gym and lifting heavy weights; sometimes just a walk in the park, gardening, housework or walking pets can suffice. Try to do at least 30 minutes of exercise every day.

TAKE A BREAK

Sometimes we all need a change of scene or a change of pace, and taking a break is really beneficial for your mental health. This could just be a five-minute timeout cleaning the kitchen, a half-hour break at lunch or getting outside for some fresh air in between meetings, but we all need time to rest. Sometimes it's good just to get away and be with your thoughts. Take a deep breath, relax and try yoga, meditation or simply putting your feet up. Often when we are trying to overachieve we work ourselves into burnout. Overworking is one of the key factors that leads to a deterioration in mental health, so it's important to never feel guilty for taking time out to do something you love or to just relax. A good tip is to remember that work is part of your life, not your life itself. During my junior doctor years, when I was working long hours way after my shift had ended, I had to remind myself that medicine wasn't my life, it was only part of my life. This way of thinking will force you to prioritise and enjoy other aspects of your life, such as socialising and exercising, even when life feels hectic and work seems like it's taking over!

BREATHE

Take a deep breath in... Now let it out. You probably feel better already, but in this section I'll give you a few tips on how to reduce stress and anxiety by doing something you do constantly, every day, and probably take no notice of... breathing!

The good thing about breathing exercises is that you can do them anywhere. Choose a place where you feel the most relaxed. If you're at home, this may be on your bed, in your living room or sitting on your work chair. You can even do these while you're out and about. Try to do them at the same time once or twice a day.

These breathing exercises can allow carbon dioxide to build up in the blood which enhances a response to the vagus nerve (a large nerve that runs through your body which is a major player for relaxation) when you exhale and stimulates the parasympathetic nervous system (the rest and digest system) to make you feel calm and relaxed. They can also regulate involuntary body functions such as temperature, help lower blood pressure and induce a sense of calm.

BELLY BREATHING

With all the hustle and bustle of life, many of us take short, shallow breaths and this can make us feel more anxious. You want to take deep breaths and really get them into your belly. This is commonly referred to as 'belly breathing'.

1. **Get comfortable: you can lie on your back with your head on a pillow or sit in a chair.**
2. **Breathe in through your nose as deeply as you can and let your belly fill with air.**
3. **Then breathe out through your nose, with one hand placed on your belly and the other on your chest.**
4. **As you breathe in through your nose, your belly should rise, and as you breathe out, your belly should lower. This is your diaphragm – the major muscle which controls breathing – contracting and relaxing.**
5. **The hand on your belly should move more than the hand on your chest.**
6. **Try to take at least three deep breaths – more if you need to – to feel really relaxed.**

AFFIRMATION BREATH FOCUS

Try to do this exercise with your eyes closed.

1. **Take a few big, deep breaths in and out.**
2. **As you breathe in, imagine the air is filled with a sense of peace and calm and feel it throughout your body.**
3. **When you breathe out, imagine the air leaving your body with stress and tension attached to it.**
4. **Use a phrase or word that helps you relax and, as you breathe, see it in your mind. Examples may include 'I breathe in peace and calm' or 'I am fully relaxed and content.'**

LION BREATHING

For this exercise, imagine that you're the king of the jungle. Yes, that's you Simba!

1. **Sit comfortably on the floor or in a chair and breathe in deeply through your nose.**
2. **Fill up your belly as much as possible with air.**
3. **When you can't breathe in anymore, open your mouth like a lion.**
4. **Then breathe out with your mouth as wide open as possible making a 'Haaa' sound.**
5. **Repeat several times until you feel less anxious or stressed and more relaxed and calm.**

BOX BREATHING

Do this breathing exercise in a stress-free, quiet environment where you can really focus on your breathing.

1. **Make sure you're seated upright in a chair with your feet flat on the floor.**
2. **Slowly exhale through your mouth, getting all the oxygen out of your lungs and focus on what you're doing to the slow count of four.**
3. **Slowly inhale through your nose, counting to four very slowly in your head.**
4. **Hold your breath for another slow count of four.**
5. **Exhale again through your mouth to the count of four, emptying the lungs completely.**
6. **Hold your breath again to the slow count of four, then repeat this process until you feel calm and relaxed.**

Create a positive mindset

Unfortunately, studies done by the NHS show that people with a more negative emotional standpoint can have weakened immune systems and may be at greater risk of illness, which is why a positive mood and mindset are so important for good health care – a poor mindset can actually leave you exhausted and lead to premature ageing.

It's said that up to 60–70 per cent of disease can be directly or indirectly as a result of stress manifesting itself. So it's important to do what you can to reduce stress and therefore reduce your risk of long-term physical disease. This comes down to purposeful positivity. We need to be careful about how we perceive our thoughts and start focusing on all the amazing things and goals that we want to achieve in life and put our energy towards that, rather than to what we fear, what may go wrong and what we don't want to have. This is one of the paths to self-improvement that can sometimes require tremendous effort. It can be hard to envision success when in reality things and situations may not be going our way. Automatically our minds can wander to negative thoughts and feelings. However, it's so important to direct our thoughts to positive affirmations, self-love and restoring our health. This is going to make us a lot happier in the long run. We need to assure ourselves that purposeful positivity will lead to manifestation of success, pleasure, love and abundance in all areas of our lives. We need to express gratitude, track our energy, value our relationships and enhance our perceptions and inspirations when it comes to positive things so we can attract good health, wealth and love.

Happiness isn't about your current situation; it isn't about the people you have around you; and it isn't even about the possessions you have. Happiness is about your own personal state of mind. These things can affect you, but only you will decide how happy you are. Don't let anyone affect your mood, but let your mood effect everyone... Good vibes only!

One-minute health hack

BE GRATEFUL

Take one minute each morning to say out loud three things you're grateful for, and watch your mindset change in just one week. For example, 'I'm grateful for my loving family. I'm grateful to have food on my table every night. I'm grateful to wake up in my own bed pain-free every day.' (See page 23 for more examples.)

Boost your self-esteem

During my time at university, I took on fitness and commercial modelling. My excitement for fashion and modelling was personal to me as I've always loved fashion. However, that's not to say that looks equal confidence and there are many other ways to feel happy and confident within yourself, and this is what I want to chat about here.

We all have times when we lack confidence and self-esteem. When we have high self-esteem it's so much easier to deal with life's ups and downs, and when it's low, life can seem like one big challenge. There are a number of health benefits that can be linked with high self-esteem and feeling and looking good. How you feel about yourself is strongly related to your mood, which then goes on to have a big impact on chronic mental health, and having good self-esteem is a big part of limiting and combatting diseases such as depression and anxiety.

Our self-esteem begins in early childhood – at school when we are with our friends, at home with family and at social activities. We build a perception of ourselves based on how we are seen in the environment and how the people closest to us react to us. The media also plays a big part in how we see ourselves, because it influences what the general perception of liked and loved people look and act like. Encouragement at a young age in schools and in the home is imperative for children's development and their self-esteem in later life. Low self-esteem can lead to people hiding away from situations and not trying new things. This can contribute chronically to depression and anxiety and other poor mental health outcomes. Loss of esteem could also lead to risky behaviour such as chronic smoking, drinking or drug abuse as a way of coping.

I remember a time – not so long ago – when I was just a young junior doctor in his first year who was told he 'dresses up too much, is too extra and wears clothes that are too tight'. Trust me, I've heard it all – from colleagues, seniors and patients alike. But at the end of the day, I wasn't hurting anyone; I was fulfilling my role as a doctor and, just as importantly, I was doing what made me feel good and what made me happy. You see, when you are more concerned about your own happiness than the opinions of others, you're able to live stress-free and fully excel in areas that give you joy. Your happiness is always most important, and prioritising it will lead to positive outcomes! Your mindset is the only thing holding you back and if you change that you truly will change your life. So go out there today, with every bit of confidence that you can be and have anything you want in this life!

HOW TO RAISE YOUR SELF-ESTEEM

In order to raise your self-esteem you need to identify the negative beliefs you have about yourself and change them. You might think you're too stupid to do something if you fail a test in class for example. Or you might consider yourself weak if you go to the gym and you see people lifting heavier weights than you. Keep a note of all these thoughts. Maybe even write them down or type them up. Then go through each one and identify when you first started to think that thought and why. Challenge these negative beliefs and try to overturn them. Write down all the positive things you think about yourself, or anything that anyone's ever told you, for example that you're a good cook or that you're a very selfless and generous friend. Aim to have 5–10 positive things on your list and update them regularly any time you think something positive about yourself or someone says something good about you.

THERE ARE PLENTY OF WAYS TO RAISE YOUR SELF-ESTEEM, INCLUDING:

- Recognising the things that you are good at: if you have a particular skill or enthusiasm for a certain topic, try to focus on it and improve and get better at it.
- Building good relationships with people who spread positivity and optimism: it's important that you surround yourself with people who are going to uplift you, not bring you down.
- Being kind to yourself: this could be in the form of saying no to things you don't want to do. People with low self-esteem can get exploited or used and feel the need to constantly people-please, even if it's to the detriment of their own health. Sometimes it's important to prioritise yourself physically and mentally.

SAFE GUARDING YOUR MIND:

A present to your future self

'

Good mental health is not a destination, but a continuous journey. Many of us strive to get better overnight, but remember it's really not about where you're going, but far more about how you drive.

'

Mental health problems are more common than we think. Approximately 25 per cent of people in the UK over the age of 16 will experience a mental health problem of some sort during their lifetime. So look at three of your friends. If it's not them, it could well be you. Twenty per cent of people in the UK report suicidal thoughts at some point and only 12.5 per cent are receiving treatment. This is why it's so important to get our mental health in order while we can. With the rise of social media, changes in our working environments and the prevalence and accessibility of alcohol and recreational drugs, mental health disorders are rising.

THE INFLUENCE OF SOCIAL MEDIA ON MENTAL HEALTH

Chances are, if you're like me, you probably really enjoy social media. Facebook, Twitter, Instagram, TikTok... they're so much fun, right? Social media is pretty ingrained into people's daily lives – so many people today are almost glued to their smartphones and have them as virtual companions. For many reasons, social media is really great – it allows us to communicate with friends and family, keep up to date with our favourite celebrities and global events, express ourselves, share ideas, thoughts and information, and promote different brands. But, unfortunately, there's also a dark side, and this relates to the impact it can have on our mental health.

Research has shown that people who spend as much as nine hours a day on social media have an increased risk of depression, anxiety, feelings of isolation and low self-esteem, and higher suicide risk, which is sad when you think about how many young people use it.

The problem is that, for so many people, social media triggers feelings of inadequacy, and because people feel as though their lives and appearance may not compare favourably with what they're seeing on social media – from their peers and from celebrities – it leads to feelings of envy and dissatisfaction. It's also said that, although you can connect with many people around the world through social media, you actually feel an increased sense of loneliness when using it. In addition, social media can facilitate cyberbullying and create an unhealthy self-centredness. Long-term use of social media throughout the day can also limit how much you're exercising and how well you're eating, and lead to low-quality sleep. This will all have an indirect consequence on your mental health.

WATCH OUT FOR SNAKE OIL PUSHERS!

When it comes to social media, it could be the best tool you've ever found or it could be your downfall depending on who you're listening to, what you're reading and where your information comes from. It's so important, especially when talking about healthcare, that we get our information from reputable government-approved sources such as the NHS or gov.uk. If you're listening to a health professional on social media, make sure they are accredited and try to ask yourself why they're saying the things they're saying and what their agenda might be. It's very dangerous to get your medical information from random and unaccredited people and sites online – this could have a big impact on the decisions you make about your health, for example whether to get a potentially life-saving vaccine or not.

Social media can be so positive and so beneficial for many of us when used in the correct way. A good tip is knowing how much you are using social media and monitoring your screen time. If you feel like you're neglecting things that matter in your life, such as personal relationships, exercising and eating well, in favour of using social media, it's time to put your phone down:

- **Set some sensible daily limits and boundaries, perhaps putting your phone away an hour before bed, not checking it first thing in the morning or not getting it out when at the table with friends or family. There are lots of good apps out there that can help you to track your screen time.**
- **Have some down time when your phone is turned off, such as when you're out with friends, spending time with the kids or driving.**
- **Unfollow accounts that have a negative impact on you and your feelings, and instead use social media to connect with those that inspire you.**
- **Turn off all those distracting notifications so your attention isn't constantly drawn to your phone.**
- **Delete some social media apps from your phone and see how you get on without them. You might find that you don't even miss them and you have time for other things like catching up with that box set or connecting with offline friends!**
- **Know when it's time to disconnect – this could be when you feel upset by a post, start to compare yourself to others or get that dreaded FOMO. Step away from the socials for a while! When you feel things are back on track, you can gradually return to using social media sensibly.**

What can I ask doctors on social media?

Along with many other doctors on social media, I get a number of people asking me for medical advice. A lot of people don't realise that doctors registered with the General Medical Council are not able to give specific medical advice to people online. To make an accurate diagnosis and give advice doctors need to be able to take a full medical history and often carry out an examination of the patient. There are specific websites and services, as well as GP practices, which allow doctors to treat you remotely; however, these are not on social media. If you're looking for medical advice you should seek advice from your GP or call 111, or 999 in an emergency.

Combatting stress

Sometimes stress can slowly creep up on us... the irony is that we are often so busy being stressed to actually realise we are! Stress and anxiety can manifest in a number of different ways:

- **increasing headaches**
- **poor sleep**
- **irritability and getting agitated**
- **stomach upset**
- **palpitations and chest pains**
- **changing eating habits**

It's important to recognise the signs early and know when to seek help, take a step back and get your mind back in control. How about trying some of the methods below?

HOW TO REDUCE STRESS

- **Make sure you're exercising regularly**
- **Study and practise relaxation techniques**
- **Regularly engage in activities that help you relax**
- **Set realistic goals and expectations, and try not to compare yourself with others**
- **When you feel anxious and stressed, make sure to take a break**
- **Identify your triggers for stress and avoid them**
- **Eat and drink healthier foods**
- **Stay organised to stop yourself from getting overwhelmed**

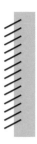

Medical myth

YOU ONLY NEED TO TAKE CARE AND BE AWARE OF YOUR MENTAL HEALTH IF YOU SUFFER FROM A CONDITION

This isn't true – we can all really benefit from making sure our mental health is in check and taking active steps to optimise it, alongside our physical health.

Dealing with depression

We all go through periods of feeling low at times; however, when you're depressed, this is classed as a psychiatric disorder characterised by persistent sadness on most days and a lack of excitement and pleasure in activities you would normally expect to enjoy.

Depression affects many of us – actually more than 300 million people worldwide – and although it's not a disease you can see, it is a debilitating one. In the UK annually 5 per cent of adults have had a period of depression and approximately 25 per cent of women and 10 per cent of men will require treatment for depression at some stage in life.

RISK FACTORS CAN INCLUDE:

- **being female; women tend to be more affected than men**
- **having a past history of depression**
- **significant physical illness causing disability or chronic pain**
- **other mental health problems, such as schizophrenia or dementia**
- **psychosocial problems, such as divorce, unemployment or poverty**
- **a history of bullying or physical or emotional abuse**
- **homelessness, asylum-seeking or poor living conditions**

As doctors, we use specific criteria to diagnose depression. Diagnosing major depression means that the patient may have at least one of the following symptoms:

- **persistent sadness and a low mood nearly every day**
- **loss of interest and pleasure in most activities**

This can then be accompanied by a myriad of other symptoms such as:

- **fatigue and loss of energy**
- **feelings of worthlessness, excessive or inappropriate thoughts**
- **recurrent thoughts of death, suicidal thoughts or actual suicide attempts**
- **diminished thinking and concentration**
- **psychomotor agitation (restlessness) or retardation (a slowing down in thoughts and physical movements)**
- **insomnia**
- **changes in appetite or weight loss**

HOW TO RECOGNISE SUICIDAL THOUGHTS

We all know how tragic suicide can be, and often people can have suicidal thoughts without even realising it. So, here are some signs to look out for:

- **having thoughts of wanting to harm or hurt yourself because you feel you don't deserve happiness or peace**
- **engaging in risky behaviour because you don't fear the consequences**
- **feeling you have no reason to live**
- **feeling you have no support**

If you recognise any of these signs in yourself – or indeed in those close to you – the most important thing to do is to seek help. Please speak to a family member or your GP. There is plenty of help out there – the NHS has many resources for people struggling with their mental health, so please do reach out.

TAKE TIME FOR OTHERS

Try to talk to someone who seems down, crack a smile, share a joke and just do what you can to make a friend or loved one happy. You never know the silent battles people face every day or the difference you can make with small, kind gestures.

What are the best ways to support my mental health?

1. **Have a good support network to talk about your feelings with:** this can be friends, family or a network or group forum online.

2. **Find something you're good at and do it:** finding enthusiasm and raising confidence in something you enjoy – whether that's sports, music, something creative or video games – is a great way to relieve stress and raise self-esteem.

3. **Pay attention to the moment:** mindfulness is really important because it helps us eliminate the worries of the past and the future and can help relieve anxiety and stress.

A&E STORY

One day working in the emergency department I saw a
29-year-old lady who came in suffering with deteriorating
anxiety and depression resulting in severe self-harm, which
led to an overdose and suicide attempt. We went through
her clinical history after blood tests, investigations and an
array of treatment. It seemed that she had been struggling
with poor mental health for years. She was so anxious
and worried that she never actually went to see her GP.
After she had recovered physically, we referred her for
psychological help from our crisis team and it appeared
she'd been having suicidal thoughts for many months and
using coping mechanisms such as marijuana and alcohol
to try to combat what she was experiencing in her mind.

This highlighted for me how important it is that people
seek help early. Just like physical diseases such as diabetes
or high blood pressure, if left untreated mental health
issues will only get worse and worse until the presentation
which could have been prevented is ultimately the only
thing that forces people to seek medical attention.

Self-love

With all that can go wrong with our mental health, it's important that we remember just how special we are. You're unique and don't deserve to be loved only by your friends and family, but by yourself as well. It's important that we practise self-love. This is about being open and honest about our well-being, our own happiness and knowing ourselves the best we can.

When you know yourself really well – inside and out – you can know what works for you health-wise. Here are some tips you can practise every day which can help:

- **Start each day by telling yourself something positive. Say something like, 'I love how you look today'; anything that will make you smile.**
- **Feed your body with delicious food that nourishes you, and that makes you thrive and feel good.**
- **Move your wonderful body every single day and love the skin you're in.**
- **Surround yourself with people who love and encourage you to remind yourself how amazing you are.**
- **Stop comparing yourself with people you see on the internet. Your only competition is you.**
- **End any toxic relationships that make you feel less than you should.**
- **Celebrate the little wins – and pat yourself on the back every once in a while.**
- **Embrace and love all the things that make you different because that's what makes you special.**
- **Step out of your comfort zone and try something new – you never know what you can accomplish.**
- **Be patient but persistent in achieving your goals. Things take time and things will come.**
- **Follow your passions and understand what gets you excited and enthusiastic.**
- **Be mindful of what you think and feel and be careful of what you watch and listen to. Feed your mind with positive stuff which encourages you.**
- **Switch off, grab your favourite cup of tea and sit down for a few minutes, just on your own, with no TV, no social media... just you and your thoughts.**

If you practise these methods every day, you're going to see visible changes in your thinking and your mindset for the better! My goal is to come back after a 12-hour shift, whip off my scrubs and feel exactly the same way Batman feels when he comes home and takes off his suit! I'm confident enough to openly speak my goals and dreams into existence, but humble enough to know that I'm just getting started and there's a long way to go. If you're sitting there wondering whether or not you can do it... I have the answer for you: You absolutely can!

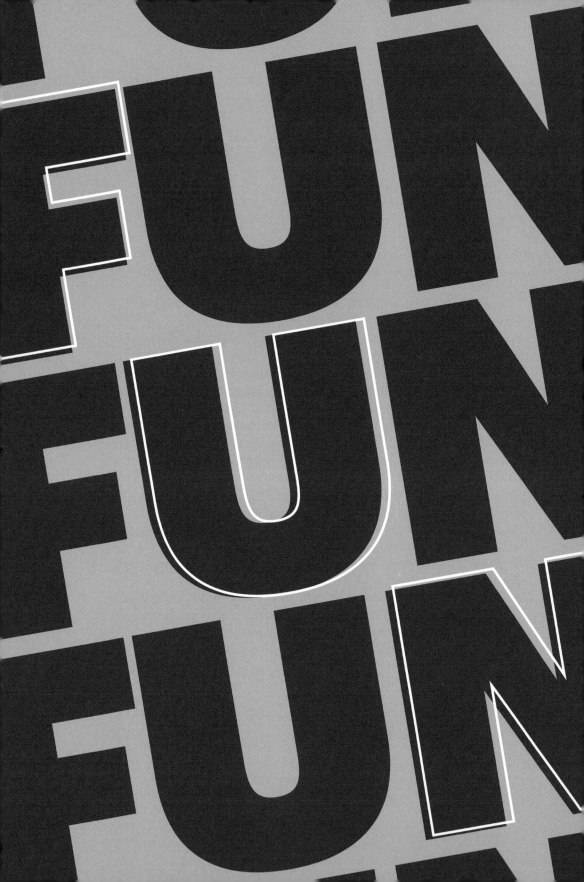

As a doctor, the more you practice, the more weird and wonderful facts you learn about the human body that many people, including myself, are sometimes very often astonished by and just can't believe... I love talking about these 'fun facts' at dinner parties and watching people's reaction to them – and I often create entertaining TikToks about them too.

Some of these facts are just general trivia; however, some of them can actually help us treat patients. I therefore thought it would be good to share some of them here with you.

Fun Medical Facts.

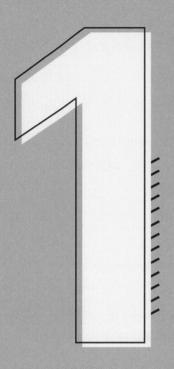

1

You are taller in the morning than the evening because the cartilage in your bones compresses throughout the day. So if you're looking for that high measurement, do it early!

2

You cannot sneeze with your eyes open.

3

Your brain replaces all of its cells every two months!

4

The largest bone in your body is your femur – the thigh bone.

More than half the bones in the human body are located in the hands, wrists, feet and ankles.

 A fully grown adult has 206 bones, but as babies we are actually born with 300 and some of them fuse together.

 Depending on the size of the person, there are between 60,000 and 200,000 miles of blood vessels in the body and if you took them out of the body you could stretch them around the world up to three times.

 Our brain uses about 20% of our oxygen and blood, and yet it only counts for 2 per cent of our body mass.

 About 60% of our body weight is made up of water. That's why you have to make sure you stay adequately hydrated.

 Pound for pound, our bones are actually stronger than steel!

11 On average, your heart beats about 100,000 times a day, sending 2 gallons of blood around your body.

12 Every year on average you produce enough saliva to fill two bathtubs! What a salivating fact!

13 The average person dreams in colour, but it's said that 12% of the population actually dream in black-and-white. Now that's old-school!

14 The average human has over 3,000 taste buds, and what's more, they're not all in your mouth – some are at the back of your throat and even in your nose.

15 Your strongest muscle isn't in your leg or even in your arms, but pound for pound it is your masseter in your jaw.

16 Our skin repairs itself every 28 days and it has about 1,000 types of different bacteria living on it.

17 On average, people produce enough gas every day to fill a party balloon!

18 The body has over 2 million sweat pores.

19 On average, people produce enough pee every month to fill a bathtub!

20 On average, we blink about 20 times a minute – that's 10 million times per year.

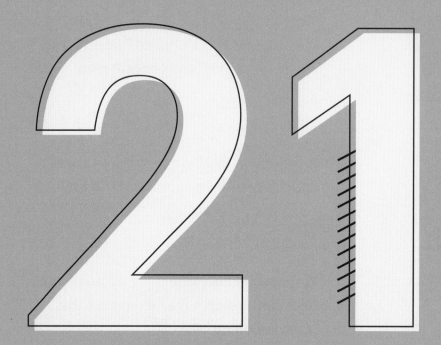

21

The cornea on your eyes is the only part of the body that doesn't have a blood supply – it gets oxygen naturally from the air.

22

Your brain can survive 5–10 minutes without oxygen.

23

However, in extreme cases of starvation, the brain will actually eat itself.

24

We spend 10% of our time awake blinking. Wow!

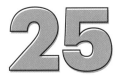 **25** We not only have unique fingerprints, but we all have a unique tongue print too.

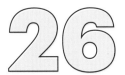 **26** We all have our own individual scent... apart from identical twins who have the same.

27 You can't tickle yourself because your brain anticipates it and defeats the surprise element.

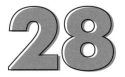 **28** You can't physically breathe and swallow at the same time. It's one or the other!

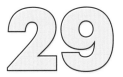 **29** On average women's brains actually shrink during pregnancy.

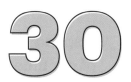 **30** Stomach acid is strong enough to dissolve some metals.

31 The human head remains conscious for 10 seconds after decapitation. Yikes!

32 The largest cell in the female body is the egg.

33 The human heart can actually beat outside of the body!

34 The human heart creates enough pressure to squirt blood 9 metres.

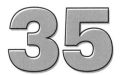 **Your tooth is the only part of your body that can't actually repair itself. You'd better get yourself a good dentist!**

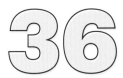 **Your nose can actually remember over 50,000 different scents.**

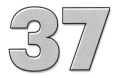 **The smallest cell in the male body is the sperm.**

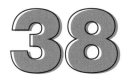 **The soles of your feet contain more sweat glands per inch than anywhere else on your body.**

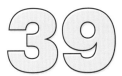 **The body contains 30,000 billion red blood cells with an average lifespan of 120 days!**

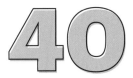 **The average adult small intestine is 7 metres long.**

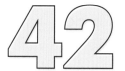 **When listening to music, at times your heart will be in sync with the rhythm.**

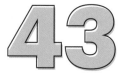 **Your ears and nose never actually stop growing throughout adulthood.**

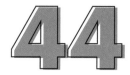 **The brain is remarkable and while you are awake it actually produces enough electricity to power a lightbulb.**

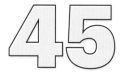 **Sexual intercourse only burns on average 3.6 calories per minute. So don't count that as your daily exercise!**

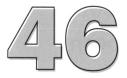 **Your body gives off enough heat in half an hour to bring over 2 litres of water to boiling point!**

One in 20 people are born with an extra rib – so instead of the usual 12 they have 13. Most people with an extra rib tend to be male.

47

One in every 2,000 babies is actually born with a tooth.

48

We share 98.4% of our DNA with chimpanzees.

49

50% of your hand grip strength comes from your pinky finger.

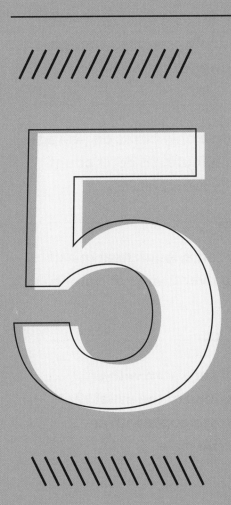

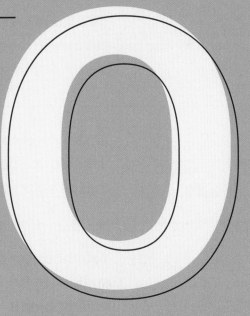

The testicles hang below the body because sperm actually dies at body temperature.

CONCLUSION

MOTIVATION

Let your rise fuel your
inspiration, your dreams push
your determination and show
the world just what you can do –
let that be your motivation.

In writing this book, my aim has been to help everyone adopt a healthier lifestyle by providing the tools and knowledge which I've shared with friends, colleagues and patients over the years, and which have benefited me throughout my life.

My aim is to inspire confidence in you, by encouraging you to follow simple health and diet hacks so you can maintain optimum health, and feel and look good at the same time, and also to remind you of why your health is so important, and what can go wrong when it's neglected.

I want you to use this book as a manual that you can always refer back to in order to keep your health in check. I want you to see just how important things like gut health and mental health are – as these are key factors in achieving good overall health for life.

Medicine has always been one of my passions. And I'm just so glad that I can try to use my enthusiasm and passion for health, fitness and nutrition to impart some of the knowledge that I have gained about healthcare to give back to others. I've always been very vocal about my future aspirations to go back to work for a charity in Nigeria and make a change. I feel I've been very fortunate with the life I've been given, and I want to make sure that I use that fortune and the position I'm in to help make a difference.

Many people go through life never knowing what their purpose is. However, I feel I know mine both as a person and as a doctor. I'm hoping that if I can go back to my birthplace and make changes it will inspire others to do the same, no matter what field they work in.

The main values I want you to take from this book are just how important healthcare is and how we all have an individual responsibility for trying to be the healthiest we can be. Here in the UK we are very fortunate to have free healthcare at the point of access. We have one of the greatest diverse health institutions in the world, made unique and irreplaceable due to the staff and patients alike. There are so many useful services the NHS provides at various levels – from primary to secondary to tertiary care. However, I'm sure most people would agree that, as great as our NHS may be, we probably wouldn't lose any sleep if we never had to go into a hospital for an emergency and would much prefer seeing the doctor only for routine check-ups and screening tests rather than for symptomatic treatment. That's what this book is for – to try to make that dream a reality!

I can't emphasise enough how daily personal healthcare should play a big part in our lives. If you're not healthy, it's harder to have a good life. You don't have to be a doctor to be able to take care of yourself. It's better for you and your loved ones if you do everything you can to keep healthy and happy for as long as possible. I am hoping that everyone reading this straightforward, practical guide, filled with simple hacks and facts about our bodies and healthcare, will now be armed with the vital information they need to help them lead healthier, happier and longer lives.

Your health now truly is in your hands.

Index

Notes

DR. EMEKA'S MINUTES THAT MATTER: THE MORNING ROUTINE

Chowdhury, M. R., 7 Dec. 2021. The neuroscience of gratitude and how it affects anxiety and grief. PositivePsychology.com. Retrieved from https://positivepsychology.com/neuroscience-of-gratitude/.

Roszak Burton, L., n.d. The neuroscience of gratitude. Wharton Alumni Club. Retrieved from https://www.whartonhealthcare.org/the_neuroscience_of_gratitude.

HOW TO LIVE LONGER: THE BASICS REVISITED

American Cancer Society, 9 Jun. 2020. Alcohol use and cancer. Retrieved from https://www.cancer.org/cancer/cancer-causes/diet-physical-activity/alcohol-use-and-cancer.html.

Ansorge, R., 15 Jan. 2020. Alcohol and medication interactions. WebMD. Retrieved from https://www.webmd.com/mental-health/addiction/alcohol-interactions-with-medications.

Division of Population Health, National Center for Chronic Disease Prevention and Health Promotion, 30 Dec. 2019. Alcohol use basics. Centers for Disease Control and Prevention. Retrieved from https://www.cdc.gov/alcohol/fact-sheets.htm.

Drinkaware, 28 Oct. 2021. Can I drive the morning after drinking alcohol? Retrieved from https://www.drinkaware.co.uk/facts/alcohol-and-the-law/can-i-drive-the-morning-after-drinking-alcohol.

Harvard Health Publishing, 6 Jul. 2020. Does cracking knuckles cause arthritis? Retrieved from https://www.health.harvard.edu/pain/does-knuckle-cracking-cause-arthritis.

Luton Council, 2020. How long does alcohol take to leave my body? Retrieved from https://m.luton.gov.uk/Page/Show/Transport_and_streets/Road_safety/Driving/Advice/Pages/How%20long%20does%20alcohol%20take%20to%20leave%20my%20body_.aspx.

Medic, G., Wille, M. and Hemels, M. E., 2017. Short- and long-term health consequences of sleep disruption. *Nature and Science of Sleep*, 9, p. 151.

National Institute on Alcohol and Abuse and Alcoholism, Jun. 2021. Alcohol facts and statistics. Retrieved from https://www.niaaa.nih.gov/publications/brochures-and-fact-sheets/alcohol-facts-and-statistics.

NHS, n.d. Quit smoking. Retrieved from https://www.nhs.uk/better-health/quit-smoking/.

Office for National Statistics, 7 Jul. 2020. Adult smoking habits in the UK: 2019. Retrieved from https://www.ons.gov.uk/peoplepopulationandcommunity/healthandsocialcare/healthandlifeexpectancies/bulletins/adultsmokinghabitsingreatbritain/2019.

Robinson, L. and Smith, M., Oct. 2021. Social media and mental health. HelpGuide. Retrieved from https://www.helpguide.org/articles/mental-health/social-media-and-mental-health.htm.

Robinson, L., Smith, M. and Segal, J., Oct. 2021. Dual diagnosis: Substance abuse and mental health. HelpGuide. Retrieved from https://www.helpguide.org/articles/addictions/substance-abuse-and-mental-health.htm.

Saitz, R., Larson, M. J., LaBelle, C., Richardson, J. and Samet, J. H., 2008. The case for chronic disease management for addiction. *Journal of Addiction Medicine*, 2(2), p. 55.

GETTING THAT BODY IN ORDER

American Stroke Association, n.d. Stroke symptoms. Retrieved from https://www.stroke.org/en/about-stroke/stroke-symptoms.

Asthma UK, n.d. Asthma facts and statistics. Retrieved from https://www.asthma.org.uk/about/media/facts-and-statistics/.

Bowel Cancer UK, Jun. 2019. Bowel cancer. Retrieved from https://www.bowelcanceruk.org.uk/about-bowel-cancer/bowel-cancer/.

Breast Cancer Now, 2021. Facts and statistics 2021. Retrieved from https://breastcancernow.org/about-us/media/facts-statistics#how%20many%20people%20die.

British Heart Foundation, Oct. 2021. Facts and figures. Retrieved from https://www.bhf.org.uk/what-we-do/news-from-the-bhf/contact-the-press-office/facts-and-figures.

British Heart Foundation, n.d. High blood pressure. Retrieved from https://www.bhf.org.uk/informationsupport/risk-factors/high-blood-pressure.

British Heart Foundation, n.d. Why should you have your cholesterol levels tested? Retrieved from https://www.bhf.org.uk/informationsupport/heart-matters-magazine/medical/tests/blood-cholesterol.

British Lung Foundation, Apr. 2020. Asthma. Retrieved from https://www.blf.org.uk/support-for-you/asthma.

British Snoring and Sleep Apnoea Association, n.d. What can I do to stop snoring? Retrieved from https://britishsnoring.co.uk/snoring/what_can_i_do_to_stop_snoring.php.

Cancer Research UK, 27 Jul. 2018. Bowel cancer. Retrieved from https://www.cancerresearchuk.org/about-cancer/bowel-cancer.

Cancer Research UK, 12 Mar. 2021. Breast cancer. Retrieved from https://www.cancerresearchuk.org/about-cancer/breast-cancer.

Cancer Research UK, n.d. Breast cancer statistics. Retrieved from https://www.cancerresearchuk.org/health-professional/cancer-statistics/statistics-by-cancer-type/breast-cancer#heading-Two.

Cancer Research UK, 19 Dec. 2019. Lung cancer. Retrieved from https://www.cancerresearchuk.org/about-cancer/lung-cancer.

Cancer Research UK, n.d. Lung cancer statistics. Retrieved from https://www.cancerresearchuk.org/health-professional/cancer-statistics/statistics-by-cancer-type/lung-cancer.

Cancer Research UK, 22 May 2019. Prostate cancer. Retrieved from https://www.cancerresearchuk.org/about-cancer/prostate-cancer.

Cirino, E., 7 Mar. 2019. 15 remedies that will stop snoring. Healthline. Retrieved from https://www.healthline.com/health/snoring-remedies.

Dinh, Q. Q. and Sinclair, R., 2007. Female pattern hair loss: Current treatment concepts. *Clinical Interventions in Aging*, 2(2), p. 189.

Knott, L., 15 Dec. 2020. Acute myocardial infarction. Patient.info. Retrieved from https://patient.info/doctor/acute-myocardial-infarction.

Mayo Clinic, 22 Dec. 2017. Snoring. Retrieved from https://www.mayoclinic.org/diseases-conditions/snoring/diagnosis-treatment/drc-20377701.

Mayo Clinic, 23 Apr. 2021. Urinary tract infection (UTI). Retrieved from https://www.mayoclinic.org/diseases-conditions/urinary-tract-infection/symptoms-causes/syc-20353447.

Mind, Feb. 2019. Seasonal affective disorder (SAD). Retrieved from https://www.mind.org.uk/information-support/types-of-mental-health-problems/seasonal-affective-disorder-sad/about-sad/.

National Institute for Health and Care Excellence, Nov. 2020. Diabetes – type 1. Retrieved from https://cks.nice.org.uk/topics/diabetes-type-1/.

National Institute for Health and Care Excellence, Nov. 2021. Diabetes – type 2. Retrieved from https://cks.nice.org.uk/topics/diabetes-type-2/.

NHS, 19 Apr. 2021. Asthma. Retrieved from https://www.nhs.uk/conditions/asthma/.

NHS, 10 Oct. 2019. Bowel cancer. Retrieved from https://www.nhs.uk/conditions/bowel-cancer/.

NHS, 28 Oct. 2019. Breast cancer in women. Retrieved from https://www.nhs.uk/conditions/breast-cancer/.

NHS, 28 Nov. 2019. Heart attack. Retrieved from https://www.nhs.uk/conditions/heart-attack/.

NHS, 15 Aug. 2019. Lung cancer. Retrieved from https://www.nhs.uk/conditions/lung-cancer/.

NHS, 29 Aug. 2018. Menopause. Retrieved from https://www.nhs.uk/conditions/menopause/.

NHS, 16 May 2019. Obesity. Retrieved from https://www.nhs.uk/conditions/obesity/.

NHS, 18 Nov. 2020. Urinary tract infections (UTIs). Retrieved from https://www.nhs.uk/conditions/urinary-tract-infections-utis/.

NHS, 15 Apr. 2019. What is high cholesterol? Retrieved from https://www.nhs.uk/conditions/high-cholesterol/.

Prostate Cancer UK, Jul. 2019. About prostate cancer. Retrieved from https://prostatecanceruk.org/prostate-information/about-prostate-cancer.

Royal College of Psychiatrists, Apr. 2015. Seasonal affective disorder (SAD). Retrieved from https://www.rcpsych.ac.uk/mental-health/problems-disorders/seasonal-affective-disorder-(sad).

The King's Fund, 4 Jul. 2021. Tackling obesity: The role of the NHS in a whole-system approach. Retrieved from https://www.kingsfund.org.uk/publications/tackling-obesity-nhs.

World Health Organization, 10 Nov. 2021. Diabetes. Retrieved from https://www.who.int/news-room/fact-sheets/detail/diabetes.

World Health Organization, n.d. Diabetes. Retrieved from https://www.who.int/health-topics/diabetes#tab=tab_1.

EMBARRASSING BODIES

Atomik Research, n.d. 50% of British guys in their thirties admit they suffer from erectile problems. Retrieved from https://www.atomikresearch.co.uk/50-of-male-brits-in-their-30s-suffer-erectile-problems/.

Kirchheimer, S., 9 Nov. 2015. 11 embarrassing health conditions. AARP. Retrieved from https://www.aarp.org/health/conditions-treatments/info-08-2013/embarrassing-health-conditions.html.

National Institute of Neurological Disorders and Stroke, 9 Jun. 2021. Brain basics: Know your brain. Retrieved from https://www.ninds.nih.gov/Disorders/Patient-Caregiver-Education/Know-Your-Brain.

FACTS FOR THE FELLAS: MEN'S HEALTH

Campbell, L., 14 Sep. 2019. Why so many men avoid going to the doctor. Healthline. Retrieved from https://www.healthline.com/health-news/why-so-many-men-avoid-doctors#The-reasons-men-stay-away-from-their-doctors.

Cancer Research UK, n.d. Cancer mortality for common cancers. Retrieved from https://www.cancerresearchuk.org/health-professional/cancer-statistics/mortality/common-cancers-compared.

Cancer Research UK, n.d. Testicular cancer statistics. Retrieved from https://www.cancerresearchuk.org/health-professional/cancer-statistics/statistics-by-cancer-type/testicular-cancer.

Diabetes UK, 13 Jul. 2009. Middle-aged men twice as likely to have diabetes as women. Retrieved from https://www.diabetes.org.uk/about_us/news_landing_page/middle-aged-men-twice-as-likely-to-have-diabetes-as-women.

Ianzito, C., 6 Sep. 2019. Why men don't go to the doctor. AARP. Retrieved from https://www.aarp.org/health/healthy-living/info-2019/survey-men-avoiding-doctors.html#:~:text=Common%20reasons%20included%20embarrassment%20or,t%20want%20to%20be%20judged.

Kautzky-Willer, A., Harreiter, J. and Pacini, G., 2016. Sex and gender differences in risk, pathophysiology and complications of type 2 diabetes mellitus. *Endocrine Reviews*, 37(3), pp. 278–316.

Mental Health Foundation, 1 Oct. 2021. Men and mental health. Retrieved from https://www.mentalhealth.org.uk/a-to-z/m/men-and-mental-health.

NHS, 14 Jun. 2019. Testicular cancer. Retrieved from https://www.nhs.uk/conditions/testicular-cancer/.

Office for National Statistics, 7 Sep. 2021. Suicides in England and Wales: 2020 registrations. Retrieved from https://www.ons.gov.uk/peoplepopulationandcommunity/birthsdeathsandmarriages/deaths/bulletins/suicidesintheunitedkingdom/2020registrations.

Pharmacy Magazine, 18 Nov. 2021 Why aren't men listening when it comes to their health? Retrieved from https://www.pharmacymagazine.co.uk/clinical/why-arent-men-listening-when-it-comes-to-their-health.

THE LOWDOWN FOR THE LASSES: WOMEN'S HEALTH

Cohut, M., 13 Jun. 2019. Women are better than men at remembering words and faces. Medical News Today. Retrieved from https://www.medicalnewstoday.com/articles/325457#Episodic-memory-in-women-vs.-men.

Loprinzi, P. D. and Frith, E., 2018. The role of sex in memory function: Considerations and recommendations in the context of exercise. *Journal of Clinical Medicine*, 7(6), p. 132.

Mental Health Foundation, 12 Oct. 2021. Women and mental health. Retrieved from https://www.mentalhealth.org.uk/a-to-z/w/women-and-mental-health.

Mind, Jun. 2020. Mental health facts and statistics. Retrieved from https://www.mind.org.uk/information-support/types-of-mental-health-problems/statistics-and-facts-about-mental-health/how-common-are-mental-health-problems/.

NHS, 4 Sep. 2018. How long does it usually take to get pregnant? Retrieved from https://www.nhs.uk/pregnancy/trying-for-a-baby/how-long-it-takes-to-get-pregnant/.

NHS, 29 Aug. 2018. Symptoms: Menopause. Retrieved from https://www.nhs.uk/conditions/menopause/symptoms/.

Office on Women's Health, 1 Mar. 2019. Eating disorders. Retrieved from https://www.womenshealth.gov/mental-health/mental-health-conditions/eating-disorders.

Taneja, V., 2018. Sex hormones determine immune response. *Frontiers in Immunology*, 9, p. 1931.

SWITCH UP YOUR DIET

Centers for Disease Control and Prevention, National Center for Emerging and Zoonotic Infectious Diseases (NCEZID) and Division of Foodborne, Waterborne and Environmental Diseases (DFWED), 11 May 2021. Key facts about food poisoning. Retrieved from https://www.cdc.gov/foodsafety/food-poisoning.html.

Guts UK!, n.d. How to increase your fibre intake. Retrieved from https://gutscharity.org.uk/advice-and-information/health-and-lifestyle/fibre/how-to-increase-your-fibre-intake/.

Harvard Health Publishing, 1 Feb. 2011. Mindful eating. Retrieved from https://www.health.harvard.edu/staying-healthy/mindful-eating.

Huizen, J., 28 Jun. 2018. Can water help you lose weight? Medical News Today. Retrieved from https://www.medicalnewstoday.com/articles/306638#summary.

NHS, 16 Oct. 2020. 10 ways to prevent food poisoning. Retrieved from https://www.nhs.uk/live-well/eat-well/10-ways-to-prevent-food-poisoning/.

NHS, 2 Aug. 2018. Bodybuilding and sports supplements: The facts. Retrieved from https://www.nhs.uk/live-well/healthy-body/body-building-sports-supplements-facts/.

NHS, 7 Dec. 2020. Diarrhoea and vomiting. Retrieved from https://www.nhs.uk/conditions/diarrhoea-and-vomiting/.

NHS, 1 Aug. 2018. How to get more fibre into your diet. Retrieved from https://www.nhs.uk/live-well/eat-well/how-to-get-more-fibre-into-your-diet/.

NHS, 8 Jun. 2020. Reference intakes explained. Retrieved from https://www.nhs.uk/live-well/eat-well/what-are-reference-intakes-on-food-labels/.

NHS, 15 Mar. 2021. Salt: The facts. Retrieved from https://www.nhs.uk/live-well/eat-well/salt-nutrition/.

NHS, 14 Jul. 2020. Sugar: The facts. Retrieved from https://www.nhs.uk/live-well/eat-well/how-does-sugar-in-our-diet-affect-our-health/.

NHS, 3 Aug. 2020. Vitamins and minerals. Retrieved from https://www.nhs.uk/conditions/vitamins-and-minerals/.

NHS, 14 Feb. 2020. Vitamins, supplements and nutrition in pregnancy. Retrieved from https://www.nhs.uk/pregnancy/keeping-well/vitamins-supplements-and-nutrition/.

Popkin, B. M., D'Anci, K. E. and Rosenberg, I. H., 2010. Water, hydration, and health. Nutrition Reviews, 68(8), pp. 439–58.

Zheng, Y., Li, Y., Satija, A., Pan, A., Sotos-Prieto, M., Rimm, E., Willett, W. C. and Hu, F. B., 2019. Association of changes in red meat consumption with total and cause specific mortality among US women and men: Two prospective cohort studies. BMJ, 365.

THAT GUT FEELING

Eske, J., 23 Oct. 2018. What's the link between cold weather and the common cold? Medical News Today. Retrieved from https://www.medicalnewstoday.com/articles/323431#rhinoviruses-and-the-common-cold.

Paoli, A., Tinsley, G., Bianco, A. and Moro, T., 2019. The influence of meal frequency and timing on health in humans: The role of fasting. Nutrients, 11(4), p. 719.

Warburton, D. E., Nicol, C. W. and Bredin, S. S., 2006. Health benefits of physical activity: The evidence. CMAJ, 174(6), pp. 801–9.

DR. EMEKA'S MINUTES THAT MATTER: THE LUNCHTIME SLUMP

Holland, K., 19 May 2019. Here's the exact number of cups of coffee you can drink per day. Healthline. Retrieved from https://www.healthline.com/health-news/6-cups-of-coffee-a-day-is-safe-but-more-isnt-healthy#What-are-the-health-benefits-associated-with-coffee-consumption?.

Lewin, J., 12 Jul. 2017. How much caffeine should I drink? BBC Good Food. Retrieved from https://www.bbcgoodfood.com/howto/guide/spotlight-caffeine.

National Institute of Diabetes and Digestive and Kidney Diseases, Feb. 2018. Health risks of overweight and obesity. Retrieved from https://www.niddk.nih.gov/health-information/weight-management/adult-overweight-obesity/health-risks.

Pandya, A. and Lodha, P., 2021. Social connectedness, excessive screen time during COVID-19 and mental health: A review of current evidence. Frontiers in Human Dynamics, p. 45.

EASY WAYS TO ADD MOVEMENT INTO YOUR DAY

Division of Nutrition, Physical Activity, and Obesity, 7 Oct. 2020. How much physical activity do adults need? National Center for Chronic Disease Prevention and Health Promotion. Retrieved from https://www.cdc.gov/physicalactivity/basics/adults/index.htm.

Sacks, R., 25 Oct. 2018. Coronary heart disease remains second leading cause of death in England and Wales. British Heart Foundation. Retrieved from https://www.bhf.org.uk/what-we-do/news-from-the-bhf/news-archive/2018/october/coronary-heart-disease-remains-second-leading-cause-of-death-in-england-and-wales.

DR. EMEKA'S MINUTES THAT MATTER: THE NIGHT-TIME WIND DOWN

Cafasso, J., 8 Nov. 2021. Do binaural beats have health benefits? Healthline. Retrieved from https://www.healthline.com/health/binaural-beats.

Halperin, D., 2014. Environmental noise and sleep disturbances: A threat to health? Sleep Science, 7(4), pp. 209–12.

Johnson, J., 13 May 2018. How long does a cup of coffee keep you awake? Medical News Today. Retrieved from https://www.medicalnewstoday.com/articles/321784.

Medic, G., Wille, M. and Hemels, M. E., 2017. Short- and long-term health consequences of sleep disruption. Nature and Science of Sleep, 9, p. 151.

National Institute of General Medical Sciences, 9 Sep. 2021. Circadian rhythms. Retrieved from https://www.nigms.nih.gov/education/fact-sheets/Pages/circadian-rhythms.aspx.

Suni, E., 10 Mar. 2021. How much sleep do we really need? Sleep Foundation. Retrieved from https://www.sleepfoundation.org/how-sleep-works/how-much-sleep-do-we-really-need.

Suni, E., 3 Nov. 2020. Light and sleep. Sleep Foundation. Retrieved from https://www.sleepfoundation.org/bedroom-environment/light-and-sleep.

LOOKING AFTER YOUR MENTAL HEALTH

Gold, A., 12 Jul. 2016. Why self-esteem is important for mental health [blog]. National Alliance on Mental Illness. Retrieved from https://www.nami.org/Blogs/NAMI-Blog/July-2016/Why-Self-Esteem-Is-Important-for-Mental-Health.

Mental Health Foundation, n.d. Mental health statistics: Stress. Retrieved from https://www.mentalhealth.org.uk/statistics/mental-health-statistics-stress.

Naylor, C., Das, P., Ross, S., Honeyman, M., Thompson, J. and Gilburt, H., 2016. Bringing together physical and mental health. The King's Fund. Retrieved from https://www.kingsfund.org.uk/sites/default/files/field/field_publication_file/Bringing-together-Kings-Fund-March-2016_1.pdf.

Salleh, M. R., 2008. Life event, stress and illness. *The Malaysian Journal of Medical Sciences: MJMS*, 15(4), p. 9.

SAFEGUARDING YOUR MIND: A PRESENT TO YOUR FUTURE SELF

American Psychiatric Association, 2013. *Diagnostic and Statistical Manual of Mental Disorders: DSM-5.*

Mammoser, G., 9 Dec. 2018. The FOMO is real: How social media increases depression and loneliness. Healthline. Retrieved from https://www.healthline.com/health-news/social-media-use-increases-depression-and-loneliness.

Mental Health Foundation, n.d. Mental health statistics: Children and young people. Retrieved from https://www.mentalhealth.org.uk/statistics/mental-health-statistics-children-and-young-people.

Mind, Jun. 2020. Mental health facts and statistics. Retrieved from https://www.mind.org.uk/information-support/types-of-mental-health-problems/statistics-and-facts-about-mental-health/how-common-are-mental-health-problems/.

National Institute of Mental Health, Oct. 2021. Major depression. Retrieved from https://www.nimh.nih.gov/health/statistics/major-depression.

Willacy, H., 30 Jun. 2020. Depression. Patient.info. Retrieved from https://patient.info/mental-health/depression-leaflet.

WITH THANKS

As this is my first book, the unconditional support and guidance I've received from so many different people really does mean a lot to me. Especially after having such a busy year, this book wouldn't have been possible without the outstanding backing, encouragement and trust of my team. My family and friends and their never-ending motivation have been the fuel for this book.

Specifically, my parents Ike and Nkechi Okorocha, who have been pushing me my whole life to achieve my dreams – one being writing this book. They've been a huge source of strength and inspiration when times have been difficult, days have been long and work has been hard. They know how much this book means to me and how much healthcare, and spreading positivity and good knowledge is vital to my whole being.

I want to say a huge thank you to my two siblings, Dr. Nneka Okorocha and Kele Okorocha, whom I'm extremely close to. Being able to confide in them and rant and rave and share ideas has been incredibly useful. The fact that the three of us are in the medical field has been a great tool as we have been able to bounce ideas off each other and discuss different topics and patient treatment methods from different standpoints.

Huge thanks to all the team at Yellow Kite. I've been privileged to be able to work with Lauren Whelan and Isabel Gonzalez-Prendergast, who have been amazing and instrumental in helping this book come to life. Thank you to my editor, Julia Kellaway, for all the tireless hours she's put in, using her expertise to precisely define the format and structure of the text. Thank you to the design team – Nic&Lou – and Nassima Rothacker, for the photography, helping bring the book to life with images. Also thank you to the food and props stylists, Hanna Miller and Hannah Wilkinson, and Senior Production Controller, Diana Talyanina.

I also want to say a massive thank you to Wendy Woolfson, my manager, my agent, my dear friend. We have spent many hours burning the midnight oil together working on this book. Without her presence and organisation of my busy schedule, none of this would have been possible. From helping me juggle the busy life of medicine and media to pushing me and aiding me during the difficult times, it's safe to say that, without her guidance, writing this book would only have been a dream.

I want to dedicate this book to all the patients we treated and lost during the Covid-19 pandemic. I've been in a position where I've seen the pain that so many have felt – from the patients themselves to their families and to my colleagues. The NHS has really had to band together over the past couple of years and without the training the NHS has given me and the opportunities I've had, I wouldn't have the knowledge and resources to construct such a book. This book is my personal dedication to my colleagues and patients alike to show my gratitude to them.

And lastly and most importantly, I'd like to thank the Lord above for being my strength and my pillar throughout this journey and for all the opportunities and grace and fortune he's given me; to put me in a position where I'm able to share my knowledge and experiences with so many in the hope that they can be beneficial to everyone. I like to feel that this is my calling, my purpose to do the good works God has brought me here for.

About Doctor Emeka

Doctor Emeka Okorocha, a Nigerian Prince, is an international media medic, author and frontline NHS doctor, working in Accident and Emergency in hospitals across London and Kent.

The award-winning doctor first appeared on our TV screens on the BBC's Junior Doctors series, and is now a regular guest on TV and radio across the world, as well as writing for, and featuring in, national and international press and publications.

Doctor Emeka works with the NHS and the Government on a variety of health campaigns and is well-known for producing a variety of inspiring, educational and entertaining social media videos on physical and mental health, well-being and mythbusting, which inspired him to write *Your Health in Your Hands* – his first book.

The fun-loving and high-energy doctor, with a passion for exercise and fitness, has been named as one of the UK's top ten TikTok educators and fronted a nationwide campaign, It Starts on TikTok, appearing on billboards across the country. He is a passionate spokesperson on Black Lives Matter and his very poignant TikTok video, appealing to people to love him in his hoodie as well as in his scrubs, captured world-wide attention.

Doctor Emeka recently scooped the Black Entertainment Film Fashion Television and Arts 'Young Achiever's Award' and was named 'Young Medical Doctor of the Year' by the Creative Faith Academy Awards.

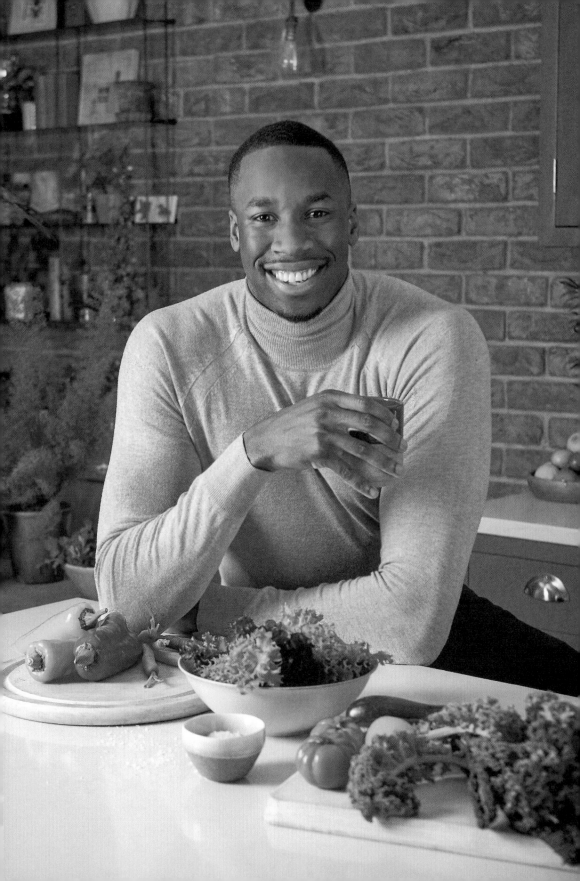

First published in Great Britain in 2022 by Yellow Kite
An imprint of Hodder & Stoughton
An Hachette UK Company

1

Hardback ISBN 9781529372533
eBook ISBN 9781529372540

Associate Publisher: Lauren Whelan
Project Editor: Isabel Gonzalez-Prendergast
Editor: Julia Kellaway
Design & Art Direction: Nic&Lou
Photography: Nassima Rothacker
Food Stylist: Hanna Miller
Props Stylist: Hannah Wilkinson
Senior Production Controller: Diana Talyanina

Colour origination by AltaImage
Printed and bound in Italy by L.E.G.O S.p.A.

Hodder & Stoughton policy is to use papers that are natural, renewable and recyclable products and made from wood grown in sustainable forests. The logging and manufacturing processes are expected to conform to the environmental regulations of the country of origin.

Yellow Kite
Hodder & Stoughton Ltd
Carmelite House
50 Victoria Embankment
London
EC4Y 0DZ

www.yellowkitebooks.co.uk
www.hodder.co.uk